VIVAS IN
GENERAL SURGERY

F.G. SMIDDY

MD, ChM, FRCS
Consultant Surgeon to the
General Infirmary at Leeds and
Clayton Hospital, Wakefield
Senior Clinical Lecturer in Surgery,
University of Leeds
Member of the Court of Examiner's of
the Royal College of Surgeons, England

GW00535860

Distributed in the USA and Canada by
BLACKWELL / YEAR BOOK MEDICAL PUBLISHERS • INC.

BLACKWELL SCIENTIFIC PUBLICATIONS

OXFORD LONDON EDINBURGH

BOSTON PALO ALTO MELBOURNE

TO MY GRANDCHILDREN

© 1987 by
Blackwell Scientific Publications
Editorial offices:
Osney Mead, Oxford OX2 0EL
(*Orders:* Tel. 0865 240201)
8 John Street, London WC1N 2ES
23 Ainslie Place, Edinburgh EH3 6AJ
52 Beacon Street, Boston
 Massachusetts 02108, USA
667 Lytton Avenue, Palo Alto
 California 94301, USA
107 Barry Street, Carlton
 Victoria 3053, Australia

First published 1987

Photoset by Enset (Photosetting),
Midsomer Norton, Bath, Avon
and printed and bound at
the Alden Press, Oxford

DISTRIBUTORS

USA
 Year Book Medical Publishers
 35 East Wacker Drive
 Chicago, Illinois 60601
 (*Orders:* Tel. 312 726-9733)

Canada
 The C.V. Mosby Company
 5240 Finch Avenue East
 Scarborough, Ontario
 (*Orders:* Tel. 416-298-1588)

Australia
 Blackwell Scientific Publications
 (Australia) Pty Ltd
 107 Barry Street
 Carlton, Victoria 3053
 (*Orders:* Tel. (03) 347 0300)

British Library
Cataloguing in Publication Data

Smiddy, F.G.
 Vivas in general surgery.
 1. Diagnosis, Surgical
 I. Title
 617'.075   RD35

 ISBN 0-632-01656-6

Contents

Preface

There are three ways in which a clinical diagnosis can be achieved: by the heuristic method in which diagnostic hypotheses are tested out one after the other, the algorithmic method in which a set pathway or series of rules are followed and thirdly, the method described as the 'fish net' approach. When using any of these different methods information must be obtained from the patient, the patient must be examined and, in the majority, investigations ordered. It has been repeatedly shown in many studies that one of the important aspects of diagnosis, if not the most important, is the collection of information from the patient. It has, for example, been demonstrated that if the facts derived from the interrogation of the patient are arranged for computer analysis the diagnostic accuracy of the interrogator himself will improve regardless of the assistance derived from the computerized database. This is, of course, merely a restatement of the classic teaching of previous generations of surgeons, to wit, that the best listeners make the best diagnosticians. Not only may valuable information be gathered by time spent listening to the patient but it also has the important additional value of making the patient feel that whoever is doing the listening is for those moments wholly absorbed in his or her problem to the exclusion of all else.

Despite efforts to introduce algorithmic methods into the diagnostic procedure, the author feels that they are doomed to failure; that whilst it may be possible to programme a computer in this way, the human mind is less disciplined and tends to arrive at a diagnosis by intuitive means; in other words the heuristic system is perhaps more natural than the more mechanical algorithmic method.

So far as the 'fish net' approach is concerned the author regards this as a method to be deplored; the excessive use of huge batteries of tests, hoping against hope that one or more will prove to be abnormal is not only expensive but also dehumanizes medicine and alienates the patient.

This book of surgical vivas, therefore, which illustrates the diagnostic and therapeutic problems associated with the surgical patient and how they may be dealt with is written using the heuristic method of approach. Although consisting of only 33 basic topics listed on p. 329 the problems associated with these patients have resulted in the consideration of several hundred different facets of surgical diagnosis and management.

Leeds 1987   F.G.S.

Acknowledgements

As with all books this book has not been written without considerable assistance and co-operation from my colleagues. It is, therefore, with gratitude that I acknowledge the assistance and advice given to me by J. Harrop Shoesmith, Lindsay Doig, John McFie and Nigel Jones, Surgeons and Paul Chennels of the Diagnostic Radiological Department at the General Infirmary, Leeds.

I should also like to acknowledge the debt I owe to the staff of the Department of Medical Photography at the Leeds Infirmary and lastly, as ever, to the devotion shown by Mrs P.M. Docherty who converted an abominable script into an acceptable manuscript suitable for submission to my publishers.

How to use this book

Within the pages of this book will be found approximately 1000 questions concerning the diagnosis and treatment of the surgical patient. One obvious method, therefore, of using the book, particularly if it is being used for the purposes of revision, is to slide a card down the text thus seeing the question before knowing the answer.

Alternatively the book can be used as a simple text book but the author feels that the first suggestion will prove more profitable to the reader.

1

A Caucasian male aged 78 was admitted complaining of difficulty in swallowing of increasing severity for two months accompanied by a weight loss of 14 pounds over a period of approximately six weeks. Only solid foods caused difficulty, liquids were swallowed without difficulty. His appetite had remained normal.

Previous medical history Five years prior to admission he had been admitted to hospital with severe melaena for which an abdominal operation had been performed.

Physical examination Essentially negative apart from a long, well healed left paramedian incision.

Question What does this history suggest.

Answer In a man of 73 with a history of progressive dysphagia over a period of two months and no prior history of dyspepsia the only reasonable presumptive diagnosis must be one of carcinoma of the oesophagus.

Question What additional symptoms may be present in carcinoma of the oesophagus.

Answer Siallorhoea and food reflux. Overspill from the oesophagus into the larynx may cause disturbed nights due to coughing, and the symptoms associated with anaemia, e.g. fatigue, lethargy and breathlessness.

Question What is the anatomical distribution of carcinoma of the oesophagus.

Answer Approximately 10 per cent occur in the upper oesophagus, i.e. from its commencement to the level of the carina or arch of the aorta. Approximately 60 per cent occur in the mid oesophagus, i.e. from the level of the carina to the inferior pulmonary ligament. Approximately 30 per cent occur in the lower oesophagus, i.e. from the level of the inferior pulmonary vein down to, and including, the gastro-oesophageal junction.

Question What investigations would you order.

Answer
1 Full blood count.
2 Upper intestinal endoscopy.
3 Ultrasound examination of the liver.
4 Barium swallow.

Question What might have been the cause of his melaena some five years previously. It appeared that he was admitted to a hospital having passed bright red blood for a period of 24 hours and that following admission the bleeding had continued with such severity that an emergency laparotomy was performed.

Answer Severe rectal bleeding in an ageing adult, in the absence of any previous intestinal symptoms and a complete absence of all physical signs, is nearly always due to diverticular disease or an angiodysplastic lesion in the colon.

Question Is massive bleeding more common in patients suffering from diverticulitis or in patients in whom asymptomatic diverticular disease is present.

Answer Severe bleeding requiring blood transfusion is much more common in the previously asymptomatic patient suffering only from diverticular disease.

Question What is the source of the bleeding in diverticular disease.

Answer Massive bleeding probably follows erosion of a peridiverticular artery.

Question What is meant by the term angioplastic lesion.

Answer Angioplasia is a condition seen in patients over the age of 60 in whom multiple small haemangiomatous lesions usually 5 mm or less in diameter develop in the caecum and ascending colon. Microscopically the veins, venules and capillaries in the submucosa and lamina propria are dilated. The great majority of such lesions are symptomless but occasionally severe bleeding occurs. These lesions are not associated with haemangiomata elsewhere. It is considered that they are the result of an ill-defined ageing process.

Question A baby presents with a massive loss of fresh blood from the anus. What is the most probable cause.

Answer Bleeding from a peptic ulcer situated in a Meckel's diverticulum in which ectopic gastric mucosa forms a part of the lining.

Question Should severe colonic bleeding occur and no abnormality is detected by double contrast barium enema what investigations might be helpful.

Answer

1 Selective arteriography. This examination is, however, only of use if bleeding in excess of 0.5 ml/min is occurring. In angiodysplasia a number of small vessels may be seen together with, in the venous phase, an enlarged vein running from the lesion. In diverticular disease only a single vessel may be seen from which leakage of contrast medium occurs and there is no enlarged draining vein.

2 Colonoscopy. Angiodysplasia on the right side of the colon may be extremely difficult to see, either because severe haemorrhage obscures vision or the lesion itself is too small. However, colonoscopy may well identify lesions which have not been seen by the radiologist, e.g. small cancers of the colon, polyps or unrecognized inflammatory disease.

2

Question What treatment has been suggested to control bleeding from an angioplastic lesion or diverticular disease.

Answer An intra-arterial injection of vasopressin, given immediately after the bleeding point is recognized by selective arteriography. This is administered at the rate of 0.3–0.6 units per minute.

Question How would you treat the patient if the colonic bleeding does not cease spontaneously or cannot be stopped by vasopressin.

Answer If the bleeding point has been recognized on colonoscopy or by selective arteriography the offending portion of the colon should be excised and the continuity of the gut restored. However, if no lesion has been positively identified the surest procedure would be total colectomy followed by an ileo-rectal anastomosis.

Question Why.

Answer Because even when left sided diverticular disease is evident an angioplastic lesion may also be present in the right colon which would be left *in situ* by performing only a limited resection of the left colon.

Comment The result of the barium swallow and ultrasound examination of the liver are shown in Figs 1.1 and 1.2.

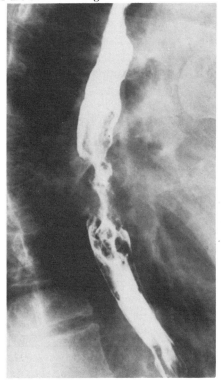

1.1

3

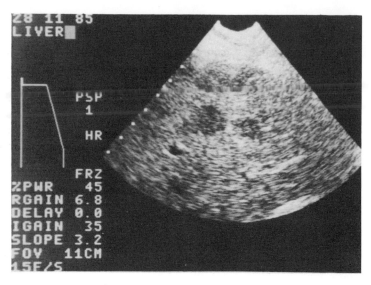

1.2

Question What does the barium swallow show.

Answer A large filling defect in the middle third of the oesophagus.

Question How much of the circumference of the oesophagus must be involved before dysphagia develops.

Answer Approximately two-thirds.

Question What is the mean delay in diagnosis in patients suffering from carcinoma of the oesophagus.

Answer Over six months.

Question What does the ultrasound examination of the liver show.

Answer Echo free areas consistent with the presence of secondary deposits in the parenchyma of the liver.

Question What further investigation would you perform.

Answer Endoscopy to establish the histological structure of the tumour.

Question What gross pathological types of oesophageal neoplasms occur.

Answer Ulcerating, lobulated, polypoid and diffuse infiltrative.

Question What histological types occur.

Answer With the exception of tumours of the cardio-oesophageal junction which are chiefly adenocarcinomata, nearly all cancers of the oesophagus are squamous tumours with varying degrees of differentiation varying from keratinizing squamous carcinomata with well formed cell nests to undifferentiated tumours without recognizable keratin or prickle cells.

Other types of primary tumour of the oesophagus which have been described include:

1 Adenosquamous tumours composed of both squamous and glandular elements.

2 Adenocarcinomata not associated with gastric neoplasms. This type of tumour has been described in all parts of the oesophagus. In some patients they occur in the absence of any abnormality of the oesophagus when they are believed to arise in the submucosal oesophageal glands. More rarely tumours of this histological structure develop in an oesophagus lined by the columnar epithelium of Barrett.

3 Carcinoma sarcoma in which both epithelial and connective tissue elements are mixed.

4 Malignant melanomata derived from melanoblasts which are rarely present in the oesophagus.

5 Carcinomata of 'oat cell', 'cylindromatous' or adenoid cystic variety can occur but are extremely rare.

Question What is the commonest type of non epithelial tumour of the oesophagus.

Answer Leiomyoma.

Question Describe the method of spread of primary oesophageal malignancy.

Answer

1 Direct spread occurs in the submucosa and submucosal lymphatics. In tumours which appear operable this feature can lead to some difficulty since submucosal extension may be present without being visible to the naked eye. A surgical purist would insist that a block should be taken from the upper line of the oesophageal resection in order to exclude involvement at the level of the anastomosis which may later lead to a recurrence at the suture line.

It should be noted that primary oesophageal carcinomata rarely extend downwards to involve the stomach.

A growth which has breached the muscle coats can involve a variety of structures including:

(a) the trachea and main bronchi.

(b) the lung parenchyma.

(c) aorta.

2 Distant spread occurs to:

(a) Lymph nodes on the parabronchial, para-oesophageal, posterior mediastinal, coeliac and lower deep cervical.

(b) Viscera, particularly the liver, lungs and adrenal glands. They occur in approximately 50 per cent of patients at the time a clinical diagnosis is made.

5

Question Have any aetiological factors been established.
Answer
>   1   Oesophageal cancer is more common in smokers and heavy drinkers than in the general population.
>   2   Carcinoma can complicate lye strictures often after a prolongod interval of time.
>   3   In the Bantu of South Africa the disease is endemic, a precise cause, however, has yet to be established.
>   4   Fe deficiency anaemia leading to the development of the Patterson-Kelly (Plumer-Vinson) Syndrome.

Question What complications may follow the development of carcinoma of the oesophagus.
Answer
>   1   Involvement of recurrent laryngeal nerve causing hoarseness.
>   2   Involvement of left bronchus producing a broncho-oesophageal fistula and copious foul smelling sputum.
>   3   Retention of food debris causing aspiration pneumonia.
>   4   Severe anaemia.

Comment The biopsy taken from this patient showed the tumour to be an adenocarcinoma.

Question How would you treat this patient.
Answer In view of the hepatic metastases any attempt at surgical excision is contraindicated. However, since the patient's chief complaint is of dysphagia an attempt to relieve this should be made.
Question When was blind peroral intubation of a malignant oesophageal stricture first attempted.
Answer In 1885 by Symonds.
Question What tubes are at present available for intubating the oesophagus.
Answer The original tube used for palliation was Soutter's tube, introduced in 1924. This has now been abandoned in favour of the Celestin or Atkinson tubes.
>   A third tube, the Moussin-Barbin tube is also available but requires a laparotomy for its insertion.
Question What is the comparative mortality between endoscopic and operative intubation.
Answer Hospital mortalities in the order of 15 per cent have been quoted in the literature for endoscopic intubation as compared to a mortality rate of twice this order for operative intubation.

Question What is the survival time of patients who are successfully intubated.

Answer Intubated patients seldom survive for longer than eighteen months.

Question What are the steps necessary prior to introducing a Celestin or Atkinson type of tube.

Answer The diagnosis is first confirmed by biopsy.

Question What does Fig. 1.3 show.

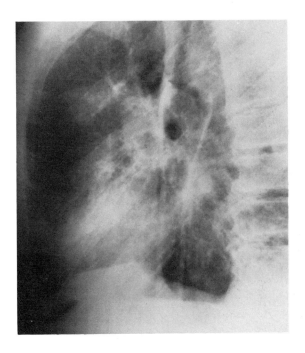

1.3

Answer A Moussin-Barbin tube within the oesophagus. Figure 1.4 shows the same tube but outlined by gastrografin, the patient having complained of retrosternal pain in the day after surgery.

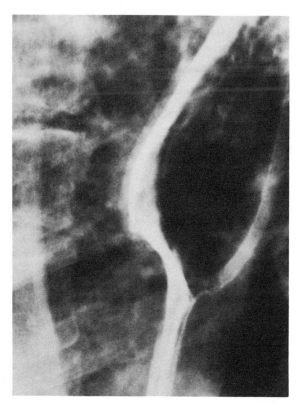

1.4

Question What are the chief complications associated with intubation.
Answer
    1 Perforation of the oesophagus leading to a mediastinitis.
    2 Proximal tube displacement, an attempt to reduce this hazard has been made by Atkinson. His tube has both proximal and distal shoulders.
    3 Blockage of the tube.
    4 Reflux oesophagitis; should the tube enter the stomach and, therefore, 'defunction' all the antireflux mechanisms.
Question What symptoms and signs would suggest a post-intubation perforation.
Answer The development of retrosternal pain and renewed dysphagia associated with a fever and possibly the development of crepitus in the suprasternal notch.

Question How would you proceed in the presence of these symptoms.

Answer

1 Forbid any further intake by mouth.

2 Order a plain X-ray of the chest.

3 Possibly order a gastrografin swallow.

Question What sign might be present on the plain X-ray.

Answer Air might be present in the mediastinum tracking upwards and downwards from the point of perforation.

Question What might appear on a gastrografin swallow.

Answer Specifically, the site of the perforation might be seen.

Question How would you treat such a case.

Answer Conservatively;

1 no fluids by mouth.

2 antibiotics, ampicillin and metranidazole.

3 intravenous fluids.

Question What advice would you give a patient in whom oesophageal intubation had been performed.

Answer

1 To sleep propped up to try and avoid reflux which can be extremely painful.

2 When eating to have a glass of soda water available in case a food particle obstructs the tube. Fish should be avoided and meat should be minced.

Question Why should an attempt be made to resect an oesophageal tumour even when the local condition suggests that the tumour is incurable.

Answer Because should the patient recover the patient has a better quality of life in that swallowing is restored to normal.

Question What are the contraindications to attempting surgical resection.

Answer Absolute contraindications include:

1 the presence of demonstrable secondary deposits in the liver or elsewhere.

2 age, patients over 75 years of age seldom survive resection.

3 tumours 7 cm or more in length. Such tumours are usually unresectable because of extensive lateral spread, in addition there may be evidence of vocal paresis or a tracheo-oesophageal fistula.

Relative contraindications include: intercurrent disease, e.g. cardiopulmonary disease which does not improve with intensive treatment and physiotherapy.

Question What is the mortality associated with resection of tumours in the mid-oesophagus.

Answer Many figures have been produced with large variations in mortality ranging from two per cent to 35 per cent. Some of this discrepancy may be due to differing operative skill but the majority must be results of case selection.

Question What are the major causes of death following oesophageal resection.

Answer Anastomotic dehiscence leading to posterior mediastinitis and pleuropulmonary complications.

Question What are the major methods now used for oesophageal resection.

Answer

1 For tumours involving the lower third of the oesophagus and cardio-oesophageal junction a left thoracotomy.

2 For tumours of the mid-oesophagus or lower part of the upper third two techniques have been described:

(a) The Ivor Lewis technique described in 1946. Basically in this approach the upper part of the stomach is first mobilized via an upper left paramedian incision after which the abdomen is closed. Two weeks later the patient is put into the left lateral position with a sandbag under the chest and the thorax is entered through the right sixth rib.

The advantages claimed for a right pleural approach are: (i) it provides for better access to the upper two-thirds of the oesophagus; (ii) only the vena azygos major needs to be divided to expose the whole length of the oesophagus; (iii) the aortic arch and to a large extent the descending aorta instead of being an obstacle becomes a safety barrier between the surgeon and the left sided mediastinal pleura.

Following mobilization of the oesophagus this viscus is divided at least 7 cm above the palpable extent of the tumour and the gastric pouch is brought up through the hiatus and the anastomosis completed.

(b) The three stage oesophagectomy as described by McKeown. This operation follows the Ivor Lewis technique in the first two steps. The stomach is mobilized by dividing: (i) the vasa brevia; (ii) the left gastroepiploic artery at the level of the lower border of the spleen; (iii) the omental branches of the left gastroepiploic artery; (iv) the left gastric artery.

This leaves the stomach supplied by the right gastric and the right gastroepiploic arteries.

Attention is then turned to the duodenum which is elevated by a radical Kocher's manoeuvre so that both the inferior vena cava and aorta are exposed over approximately 8 cm.

In the second stage the oesophagus is exposed through a right sixth rib resection and the tumour together with the whole length of the intrathoracic oesophagus is mobilized and the stomach pulled through a widened hiatus.

In the third stage a small transverse incision is made in the neck above the level of the clavicle. The cervical oesophagus is carefully separated from the trachea and the stomach is pulled into the incision. The oesophagogastric junction is divided and the fundus of the stomach is anastomosed to the cervical oesophagus.

Question What is the ultimate prognosis assuming the patient survives.

Answer According to most workers in this field only approximately five per cent of patients will live for five years. Much depends on the presence or absence of involved lymph nodes. The Japanese workers reported a 54 per cent survival for five years in the absence of lymph node involvement and a 15 per cent survival in lymph nodes were found to be involved.

Question What other alternative treatment has been described.

Answer

1 Radiotherapy. This is particularly effective in cancers occurring in the upper two-thirds of the oesophagus in which nearly all malignant disease is of the squamous variety. However, squamous carcinoma of the oesophagus is only moderately radio sensitive and rather unpredictable in its response. The Edinburgh experience quoted by Pearson in 1977 in which some 2000 patients were studied suggests that there is little to choose between the results obtained by surgery and by radiotherapy. A one year survival of 25 per cent and a five year survival of eight per cent can be achieved by radiotherapy which compares favourably with the results obtained following surgical excision.

2 The recent introduction of laser therapy into surgery means that in some cases intubation can be avoided by progressively removing the central core of the tumour using a VAG source and a flexible fibreoptic endoscope. Good results in terms of the quality of life and swallowing have been claimed by the protagonsists of this method.

2

A male aged 72 years was admitted complaining of difficulty in swallowing and loss of weight of six months duration

Physical examination This revealed a thin somewhat emaciated man, otherwise there were no positive signs.

Previous medical history Thirteen years before admission when aged 59 this man had presented in outpatients complaining of a 12 month history of epigastric discomfort, fullness after meals and recent weight loss. At that time no physical signs were present. A tentative diagnosis of gastric ulceration or carcinoma was made and a barium meal was ordered.

The results of this investigation are shown in Fig. 2.1.

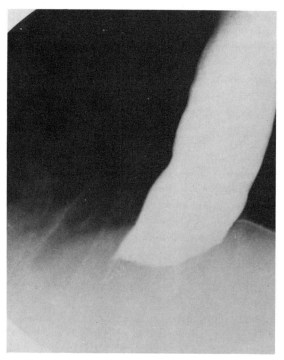

2.1

Question What are the chief radiological signs shown in this figure.
Answer Dilatation of the oesophagus with beak-like tapering of the

oesophagus at the gastro-oesophageal junction consistent with a diagnosis of achalasia.

Question What are the classic symptoms of this condition.

Answer

1 Dysphagia for both liquid and solid foods.

2 Chest discomfort or pain.

3 Spontaneous or postural regurgitation of foamy, mucoid saliva.

4 Loss of weight.

Question Is this condition more common in females than males.

Answer No, the sex incidence of this condition is approximately equal.

Question Is achalasia commonly associated with a long history.

Answer Yes. In many older patients gradually increasing dysphagia may have been present for several decades prior to the diagnosis being made.

Question In more advanced cases, illustrated in Fig. 2.2, what further radiological changes may be seen in this condition.

Answer The oesophagus may be so dilated that it assumes a sigmoid shape; an air/fluid level may be present. Also in some long standing cases, pneumonitis may be seen on the plain chest X-ray the result of spillage of the oesophageal contents into the trachea.

Question Is endoscopy necessary.

Answer Yes. Endoscopy is essential to confirm the diagnosis and eliminate carcinoma of the lower oesophagus as a cause of the symptoms and radiological appearances. Stagnation of food debris may cause oesophagitis which in severe cases may give rise to a haematemesis.

Question What clinical features differentiate achalasia from carcinoma of the oesophagus.

Answer Usually the length of the history and the rapid progression of symptoms in carcinoma of the oesophagus.

Question Who is reputed to have first treated a patient suffering from achalasia.

Answer In 1675 Thomas Willis described a patient suffering from dysphagia on whom he passed a sponge through the cardia on the end of a piece of whalebone.

Question What other investigation can be used to confirm the diagnosis.

Answer Oesophageal manometry. This is rarely used as a routine investigation. Nevertheless it is useful in distinguishing the various forms of motility disturbance which can affect the oesophagus.

Question How does oesophageal motility differ from normal in patients suffering from cardiospasm.

Answer In the normal oesophagus in the region of the hiatus an absolute rise in pressure occurs which extends over a distance of 1–4 cm,

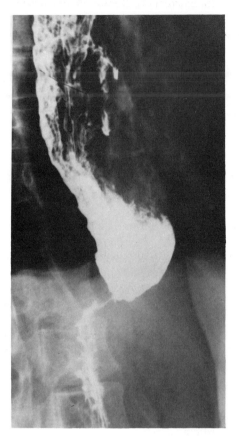

2.2

beginning 1 cm below and ending 2–3 cm above the diaphragmatic
hiatus. The high pressure zone marks the manometric position of
the lower oesophageal sphincter, a physiological rather than an
anatomical entity. Swallowing in a normal individual is followed by
a decrease in pressure in this zone, indicating that it is normally in
a state of tonic contraction. In a patient suffering from achalasia
violent waves of contraction causing peaks of high pressure occur
in the upper oesophagus on swallowing. These are less marked in
the lower oesophagus and most important of all the lower
oesophageal sphincter, i.e. the high pressure zone fails to relax, as
in a normal individual on swallowing.

Question Is muscular hypertrophy present in the affected segment of the oesophagus.

Answer No. However, hypertrophy occurs proximal to the high pressure zone in the upper oesophagus.

Question Is the condition due to spasm.

Answer No. In 1927 Hurst of Guy's Hospital established that the cause of this kind of dysphagia was failure of the affected segment of the oesophagus to relax. It was as a result of Hurst's observations that the name of the condition was altered from cardiospasm to achalasia.

Question When was the first operative treatment of this condition described.

Answer In 1913 by Heller who described the operation of cardiomyotomy although a similar solution had been suggested by Gottstein in 1901.

Question What did Heller think he was achieving.

Answer Relief of spasm at the lower end of the oesophagus, the hypothesis later disproved by Hurst.

Question Are any structural changes present in the lower end of the oesophagus.

Answer The nerve fibres and ganglia of Auerbach's plexus may be absent. In addition histological abnormalities have been demonstrated in the dorsal vagal ganglia

Question Has any pharmacological abnormality been identified.

Answer Yes. The lower oesophageal sphincter reacts strongly to cholinergic stimulation and is also supersensitive to gastrin.

Question What are the two accepted methods of treating achalasia.

Answer

1 Dilatation of the narrow segment.

2 Heller's cardiomyotomy.

Question Who first described dilatation as a method of treatment of achalasia.

Answer Russel in 1898 who used a silk covered rubber bag which could be inflated with air.

Comment Since that time a variety of devices have been used to dilate the lower end of the oesophagus and dilatation as an alternative to operative intervention has been advocated by many gastro-enterologists. In general dilatation is achieved by hydrostatic or pneumatic bags the maximal diameter of which is fixed. Various authorities differ as to the degree of dilatation required, many suggesting 3 cm as a maximum and others 4.5 cm. Whatever method is used it is essential that the balloon is positioned correctly and for this to be achieved radiological control is necessary. Dilatation may require repeating. The particular patient referred to in the history refused operative intervention and has required dilating at approximately two yearly intervals since his first attendance 13 years previously.

Question What complication may follow hydrostatic dilatation?
Answer Perforation of the oesophagus,
Question How is this complication recognized?
Answer Perforation of the oesophagus permits the leakage of air and fluid into the posterior mediastinum. This causes severe praecordial and epigastric pain together with difficulty in swallowing.
Question What physical signs may be associated with perforation of the oesophagus.
Answer
1   Tachycardia.
2   Upper abdominal rigidity.
3   Rarely surgical emphysema in the supraclavicular region.
4   The mediastinal 'crunch' sign described by Hammen; auscultation revealing a crackling sound with each heart beat when the patient holds their breath.
5   If the condition has gone unrecognized for several days percussion and auscultation may reveal the presence of a pleural effusion.
Question What investigations confirm the diagnosis.
Answer
1   PA and lateral plain chest X-rays may reveal the presence of varying quantities of air in the mediastinum, a retropharyngeal mass if the perforation is in the cervical oesophagus or a pleural effusion.
2   A gastrografin swallow demonstrates extravasation into the mediastinal tissues.
Question What are the principal causes of oesophageal perforation.
Answer
1   Instrumental perforation. Prior to the introduction of fibreoptic flexible oesophagoscopes the commonest cause of perforation of the oesophagus was the passage of a rigid oesophagoscope. Perforation could be caused either by tearing the pharynx or cervical oesophagus during the introduction of the instrument or by pressure necrosis, the instrument compressing the oesophagus against the cervical spine.
2   Non instrumental perforation.
  (a) Spontaneous perforation of the oesophagus was first described by Boerhaave in 1723. It normally occurs in an individual who raises intra-oesophageal pressure by suppressing vomiting. The perforation involves the lower end of the oesophagus and characteristically the mucosal tear is always of greater length than that in the muscular

wall, a point of great technical importance when attempting to repair the rupture.

(b) Perforation by ingested materials among which fish, chicken and rabbit bones are the most common.

(c) Penetrating injuries of the chest or neck by bullets or knife wounds.

Question How would you treat a perforation of the oesophagus.

Answer This depends upon the cause, the position of the perforation and the time interval between the event and diagnosis. The majority of instrumental perforations, excluding those caused by dilatation of cardiospasm, are high perforations involving the cervical oesophagus. These perforations are treated conservatively. Fluids and food by mouth are withheld, intravenous fluids and a broad spectrum antibiotic are administered. If an abscess forms this is drained.

Perforation of the lower oesophagus should be repaired if recognized within 24 hours. The mucosal tear must be identified along its whole length before beginning the suture of the defect. At the completion of the operation, performed via the bed of the left eighth rib, the chest is drained. If the condition is unrecognized the development of mediastinitis usually results in failure of simple suture and the condition must be managed conservatively treating the complications as they occur, e.g. a pleural effusion may respond to simple aspiration whereas an empyema may require surgical drainage.

Question What other condition may follow the suppression of vomiting.

Answer Haematemesis due to the development of the Mallory-Weiss syndrome. The Mallory-Weiss syndrome consists of mucosal tears normally involving the cardia. The condition is believed to be a cause of about eight per cent of all cases of upper gastrointestinal bleeding although it is rarely fatal. Prior to the use of fibreoptic endoscopy the condition was undiagnosed but if endoscopy is performed early the mucosal tear or tears at the cardia can be seen. It occurs in a variety of individuals including particularly alcoholics and patients in whom nausea and vomiting is being caused by treatment, e.g. chemotherapy. This condition normally settles without surgical intervention.

Question What is the overall mortality of dilatation.

Answer In a collected world series of over 2000 patients the mortality of this procedure was somewhat less than 1 in every 400 patients treated.

Question What other complication can follow dilatation.

Answer Gastro-oesophageal reflux. In a series published from John Hopkins this was detected radiologically in 17 per cent of patients but assumed serious significance in only two per cent and in none of these patients did a stricture develop.

Question What proportion of patients have a good result following dilatation.

Answer Approximately 80 per cent.

Comment In this patient symptomatic improvement together with weight gain due to an improved ability to swallow occurred after each dilatation.

Question What is Heller's operation.

Answer Cardiomyotomy. The division of the muscle fibres of the oesophagus and stomach down to mucosa from a point 5 cm above the cardia to 1 cm below.

Question Is the length and depth of the myotomy important.

Answer Yes. Too deep a myotomy causes perforation of the oesophagus. Too long an incision on the gastric side leads to reflux. To obviate the dangers of perforation the myotomy should be performed with a 5 F bougie in place.

The proposed ideal incision is one made on the lesser curve side of the oesophagus and stomach so as not to injure the oblique muscle fibres of the stomach which are one of the four major antireflux mechanisms.

Question What is the reported incidence of gastro-oesophageal reflux following Heller's operation.

Answer Approximately 10 per cent, one-third of whom are reported to develop an oesophageal stricture.

Question Can a satisfactory Heller's operation be performed via an abdominal approach.

Answer Yes.

Question What is the mortality associated with Heller's operation.

Answer Approximately one per cent.

Question What percentage of patients achieve a satisfactory result following Heller's operation.

Answer Approximately 75 per cent.

Question What is the major cause of dissatisfaction following Heller's operation.

Answer Uncontrolled reflux oesophagitis.

Comment Many papers have now been published confirming that the results of Heller's operation are greatly improved if at the same time as the cardiomyotomy an anti-reflux procedure is also performed.

3

A female aged 86 years presented in outpatients complaining of increasing dysphagia of six months duration, particularly for solid foods together with the loss of 4 kg in weight.

Past medical history 20 years previously she had complained of a sensation in her epigastrum as if she had swallowed a brick. This had been present for approximately one year and developed some 30 minutes after eating. Her additional symptoms were those of severe heartburn and acid regurgitation together with the loss of 5 kg in weight.

Question What do these symptoms suggest.
Answer The presence of gastro-oesophageal reflux.

Comment At that time a barium swallow and meal were performed and no evidence of reflux or a hiatus hernia was demonstrated. A cholecystogram performed after this negative investigation also showed no evidence of disease.

In view of the negative investigations she was treated with antacids which she took for several months.

Five years previously, i.e. 15 years after her initial presentation she had returned to outpatients complaining that for 18 months she had been suffering from a sensation of choking whilst eating, a symptom somewhat eased if she took a drink before beginning solid food. Over the same period she had noted that stooping produced praecordial discomfort and regurgitation. A constant feeling of indigestion had led to her taking large doses of bicarbonate. At that time a further barium swallow was performed the results of which are shown in Fig. 3.1.

Question What does Fig. 3.1 show.
Answer A penetrating ulcer approximately 6 cm above the cardio-oesophageal junction, a stricture approximately 2 cm in length below which is the gastric pouch of a hiatus hernia.
Question What essential investigation should now be performed.
Answer Oesophagoscopy together with multiple biopsies of the ulcerated area to establish whether this is benign or malignant.

Comment This was carried out and the biopsy material found to be benign. In view of the advanced age of the patient a decision was made to treat her conservatively. She was placed on the following

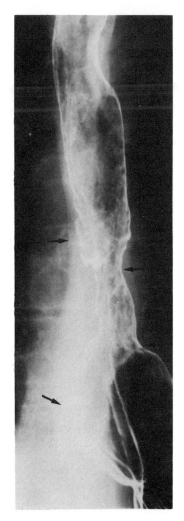

3.1

medication: Cimetidine 200 mg bd and 400 mg at night; Gaviscon (Reckitts and Coleman, UK) 2 tablets after meals and at bedtime.

Question What is the action of cimetidine.
Answer Cimetidine is an H_2 receptor antagonist, for further details see p. 68.
Question What is Gaviscon.
Answer Gaviscon tablets contain the following:
Dried aluminium hydroxide, 100 mg.

Magnesium trisilicate, 25 mg.

Alginic acid, 500 mg.

Sodium bicarbonate 170 mg.

Sucrose and mannitol.

The first two drugs are long established antacids, alginic acid in contact with fluid forms a highly viscous solution.

Question What other drugs may prove helpful in this condition.

Answer

1 Carbenoxolone (Biogastrone (Winthrop UK)), 100 mg tds. This drug should, however, be used with caution in the elderly since it causes sodium and water retention which may lead to oedema, hypertension and hypokalaemia.

2 Bethanechol chloride, 25 mg qid, this drug is a quarternary ammonium parasympathomimetic agent with the muscarinic actions of acetylcholine. Its use in this condition is based on its ability to increase the tone of the lower oesophageal sphincter.

Comment On this regime her symptoms diminished but 2 years prior to the present complaint she presented with diarrhoea of 12 weeks duration, nine weeks bleeding per rectum and the passage of much mucous. Rectal examination revealed a carcinoma of the rectum and a low anterior resection was performed. She made an uneventful recovery but was left with slight incontinence which gradually improved over the following year.

Histological examination of the tumour showed it to be a poorly differentiated adenocarcinoma, Stage C. However, no intra- or extramural lymphatic invasion was present and all nine lymph nodes examined were free from tumour.

Question What is the explanation for the increasing dysphagia noted in the six months prior to her attendance at the outpatient department.

Answer Either the development of a carcinoma of the oesophagus or increasing severity of the previously recognized oesophageal stricture.

Question What investigations are required.

Answer

1 A barium swallow is shown in Fig. 3.2.

2 Oesophagoscopy and biopsy of the stricture.

Question What does Fig. 3.2 show.

Answer No obvious oesophagitis, no apparent ulceration, the presence of an oesophageal stricture inferior to which is a large hiatus hernia.

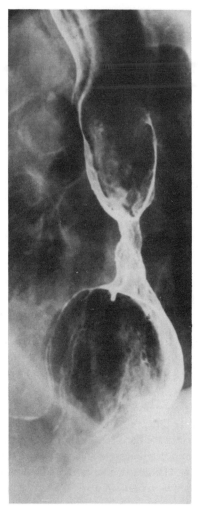

3.2

Comment Oesophagoscopy revealed:
1   Severe oesophagitis in the terminal oesophagus.
2   A benign stricture at 32–34 cm.
3   Biopsies negative for malignant disease.

Question How would you treat this patient.
Answer In view of her age the stricture was dilated using Celestin dilators.
Question What other oesophageal dilators are in use.

22

Answer
1 Chevalier Jackson's bougies, passed through a rigid oesophago-scope.

2 The Eder-Pueston dilator, these are olive-tipped metal dilators which are passed over a guide wire introduced through the stricture by means of a fibreoptic oesophagoscope.

Question What other type of stricture can occur in patients suffering from a hiatus hernia.

Answer A Schatzki ring first described by Schatzki and Gary in 1953. This type of stricture is caused by submucosal fibrosis at the squamocolumnar junction. They are seldom greater than 3 mm in length. They are nearly always associated with a hiatus hernia and the submucosal scar is presumed to be a sequel of reflux.

Comment When seen six months later the patient was free of symptoms.

Question From what type of hiatus hernia is this patient suffering.

Answer A Type I or sliding hernia.

Question What other types occur.

Answer The Type II, also known as the para-oesophageal hernia and mixed types, a combination of both.

Question What is the essential anatomical difference between the Type I and Type II hernia.

Answer In a Type I hernia the cardio-oesophageal junction, marked by the squamocolumnar junction lies above the level of the hiatus.

Question What is the essential physiological difference between the two types of hernia.

Answer The presence of the cardio-oesophageal junction above the dia-phragm in the Type I hernia may lead to gastro-oesophageal reflux.

Question What are the classic symptoms associated with a hiatus hernia accompanied by gastro-oesophageal reflux.

Answer
1 Heartburn of varying degree, aggravated by recumbency or stooping.
2 Flatulence.
3 Post-prandial fullness.
4 Dysphagia.
5 Ill-defined chest pain.

However, such symptoms may also be caused by a number of oesophageal conditions, e.g. achalasia, in abdominal conditions (e.g. choleliathiasis) and in cardiac conditions (e.g. coronary atherosclerosis).

Question What factors are believed to be responsible for cardio-oesophageal competence.

Answer

1   The physiological sphincter at the lower end of the oesophagus, a zone demonstrable by manometry but anatomically indefinable.

2   The acute angle of entry of the oesophagus into the stomach, this may be maintained by the oblique muscle fibres arising from a lesser curve. These fibres are extremely well marked in the dog but are not so obvious in the human.

3   The presence of an intra-abdominal oesophageal segment.

4   The mucosal rosette described by Botha at the gastro-oesophageal junction.

Question Can symptomatic reflux occur in the absence of a sliding type of hernia.

Answer Yes.

Question What physiological abnormalities can be demonstrated in a patient suffering from reflux.

Answer

1   The sphincteric pressure at the lower end of the oesophagus may be lowered. However, this is not necessarily so. Excessive reflux can be demonstrated in patients in whom the sphincter pressure is normal. Using a pH probe in order to document the presence or absence of gastro-oesophageal reflux over long periods Johnson and De Meester found that reflux occurred in perfectly normal individuals without any evidence of gastro-intestinal disease although these episodes of reflux were commoner during the daytime than at night. The reason that such refluxed material does not cause symptoms is because the oesophagus is rapidly cleared by swallowing and in addition partial neutralization occurs by swallowed saliva.

2   Peristaltic activity in the oesophagus may be reduced. This abnormality is clearly demonstrated in patients suffering from oesophageal scleroderma. The result of such a physiological disturbance is to reduce the ability of the oesophagus to clear itself of regurgitated acid.

De Meester and others have clearly shown that the lower oesophageal sphincter pressure can be normal in patients suffering from severe oesophagitis but oesophageal clearance is abnormal.

3   The rate of gastric emptying is slowed in patients suffering from reflux.

Question Does the severity of the symptoms in gastro-oesophageal reflux bear any relationship to the pathological changes in the wall of the oesophagus.

Answer No.

Question What are the chief pathological changes in peptic oesophagitis.

Answer In order of their appearance the chief pathological changes are as follows:

1 Hyperplasia of the basal cell layer, increasing its thickness beyond the normal 15 per cent, together with some thinning of the epithelium over the papillae.

2 Polymorphonuclear infiltration of the lamina propria.

3 Longitudinal ulceration which ends abruptly at the cardia but tails away gradually into the proximal mucosa.

4 Submucosal fibrosis of varying severity which may gradually extend outwards to involve not only the muscle coats but also the peri-oesophageal tissues.

Question In this patient the ulceration seen in Fig. 3.1 is deep and penetrating. Is this typical of the ulceration seen in the common form of reflux oesophagitis.

Answer No. This type of ulcer occurs only in areas of true gastric heterotopic epithelium, in zones of columnar cell metaplasia, or the junctional zone between the normal squamous epithelium of the oesophagus and a zone of columnar cell metaplasia.

Question How does this type of ulcer differ from the more typical superficial ulceration associated with reflux oesophagitis.

Answer This type of ulcer may be complicated by perforation and haemorrhage. Microscopically the ulcerated mucosa is replaced by granulation tissue, the muscle coat of the oesophagus is destroyed and the base is formed of fibrous tissue.

Question What was the name given to this condition when it was originally described.

Answer A Barrett's oesophagus. Barrett first described this condition in 1950. His original hypothesis was that the condition occurred in patients with a congenitally short oesophagus. However, in 1953, Allison and Johnstone postulated that the intrathoracic columnar epithelium resulted from metaplastic extension orally of the non-acid secreting columnar epithelium which lines the distal part of the normal gastro-oesophageal junction and the gastric cardia.

Question What is the frequency of Barrett's oesophagus.

Answer Approximately 4.5 per cent in patients complaining of oesophageal reflux associated with a hiatus hernia.

Question Can Barrett's columnar epithelium be distinguished from squamous epithelium.

Answer Yes, by its structure, transparency and colour. A columnar-lined oesophagus is also tube-like and lacks the folds seen in an intrathoracic stomach. In colour it is a deeper red than the normal gastric mucosa.

25

Question What is the histological structure of the epithelium distal to the stricture.

Answer A spectrum of histological patterns occurs. The first and most common is an oesophagus linea by a specialized form of columnar epithelium within which mucus secreting goblet cells and sometimes Paneth cells can be found. A second pattern is a gastric fundal type of epithelium in which both parietal and chief cells may be present and lastly, both patterns may coexist. However, in this third pattern the columnar epithelium is always oral to the gastric and there may be a junctional zone between them containing mucous glands similar to those of the cardia. In addition to these major cell types enterochromaffin, gastrin and somatostatin cells can also be found.

Question Can dysplastic changes occur in such an epithelium and, if so, what is the indication of its presence.

Answer

1   The nuclear-cytoplasmic ratio is increased.
2   Hyperchromatism with loss of polarity.
3   Pleomorphism.
4   Mitoses.
5   Marked distortion of the glandular pattern.

Question Can frank invasive malignancy occur.

Answer Yes. The fact that columnar metaplastic epithelium is liable to carcinomatous change is the indication for multiple biopsies in this condition and is a strong indication to perform an anti-reflux operation.

Question In a Barrett's oesophagus in which area does oesophagitis occur.

Answer In the squamous epithelium adjacent to the squamocolumnar junction.

Question Had this patient been younger would there have been an indication to perform an anti-reflux type of procedure.

Answer Possibly if severe symptoms of oesophagitis were present.

Question Would an anti-reflux procedure produce regression of the ectopic epithelium.

Answer Conflicting reports are recorded in the literature but on balance the evidence suggests that in the majority of patients whilst the symptoms of reflux may be diminished the ectopic epithelium remains. If dysplastic changes are already present this suggests that there is a continuing danger of frank malignancy developing.

Question What surgical anti-reflux procedures are available in patients in whom the condition is associated with a hiatus hernia.

Answer

1   The Nissen fundoplication *Schweiz. med. Wochenschr.* 1956 **86**, 590.

2 The Belsey Mark IV technique *Surgery* 1967 **62**, 396.

3 The Colliss operation *J. Thorac. Cardiovasc. Surg.* 1957 **34**, 768

4 Combined Collis/Belsey technique.

5 Combined Collis/Nissen fundoplication technique.

6 The Hill technique *World J. Surg.* 1977 **1**, 425.

These various procedures have superceded the original technique proposed by Allison which was in reality an anatomical repair in which the aim was to remove the hernial sac, reconstitute the stretched phreno-oesophageal ligament and then plicate the crura at the oesophageal hiatus.

Of the various procedures described above none are perfect, although the originators of each technique describes excellent results. Thus Hill achieved 99.2 per cent success with his median arcuate repair which anchors the gastro-oesophageal junction posteriorly whilst Belsey after operating upon 632 patients claimed that 97 per cent were improved.

However, any patient undergoing surgical correction for reflux and its complications should be warned about the possibilities of post-operative dysphagia, the 'gas bloat syndrome', post-operative gastric distension due to unplanned vagotomy, the possible failure to relieve symptoms and recurrence and lastly, the persistence of a stricture if this is present.

Comment The references above give details of the operative technique used by the various authors.

In this elderly patient it seemed reasonable in view of further negative biopsies to persist with conservative treatment. The stricture the chief cause of her dysphagia, was therefore dilated using Eder-Pueston dilators and she once again received H_2 antagonists. When last seen six months later she remained symptom-free.

4

A female, 58 years of age, was admitted complaining of severe abdominal pain and intermittent vomiting of three days duration. She described the pain as burning in character radiating from the epigastrium, to the back, retrosternally and later across the whole abdomen. The onset of the pain had been associated with the vomiting of undigested food and later brownish fluid but no recognizable fresh blood. Her bowels had not been open for three days.

Two years previously she had been investigated for a complaint of intermittent nausea associated with three attacks of severe epigastric and precordial pain. Each of these attacks had lasted approximately one hour and had been relieved by vomiting. There appeared to be no precipitating factors and no dysphagia. Her appetite had remained good. The differential diagnosis at that time had been as follows:

1 Functional dyspepsia.
2 Gall-stones.
3 Gastric ulcer.

Both endoscopy and an ultrasound examination of the upper abdomen had yielded negative results and in view of this a diagnosis of functional dyspepsia was made and the patient was reassured.

Some three months later she was again seen, stating that she had suffered a further attack of much more severe abdominal pain which had lasted for approximately two days. No physical signs were found and she was once again reassured.

One year prior to admission she had become aware of a swelling in the neck. Physical examination revealed that both thyroid lobes were enlarged, the right somewhat more than the left. The outline of the thyroid was preserved and it was of firm consistency.

Question What do the physical signs in the neck suggest.
Answer Lymphadenoid goitre.
Question Who first described lymphadenoid goitre.
Answer Hashimoto in 1912 described the distinctive histological appearance of this condition.
Question To what group of diseases does Hashimoto's disease belong.
Answer Organ specific autoimmune disease.
Question What other conditions fall into this category.
Answer Thyrotoxicosis, atrophic gastritis, pernicious anaemia and Addison's disease.

Question What are the chief characteristics of organ specific autoimmune disease.

Answer

1 The disease is much commoner in women than in men.

2 It occurs most commonly about 40 years of age.

3 There is a tendency for more than one autoimmune disorder to develop in the same individual. Thus 10 per cent of patients suffering from Hashimoto's disease suffer from coincidental pernicious anaemia as compared to 0.2 per cent of the normal population.

4 There is frequently a family history of Hashimoto's disease, primary hypothyroidism or Graves disease.

5 The serum of asymptomatic relatives in whom overt thyroid symptoms are absent may contain autoantibodies.

Question What is the gross appearance of the thyroid gland in Hashimoto's disease.

Answer The general shape of the thyroid gland is preserved although there may be unequal enlargement of the lobes. The normal lobular pattern is exaggerated and the gland appears pale and relatively avascular.

Question What are the characteristic histopathological features.

Answer The overall picture is of diffuse lymphocytic infiltration associated with destruction of the thyroid follicles and fibrosis. The follicular cells are destroyed and the follicular basement membrane fragmented. Scattered within the thyroid are larger cells showing oxyphilic changes in the cytoplasm. These are the Askanazy cells which are pathognomonic of this disease. Typical lymphoid follicles within which are germinal centres are normally present.

Question What physiopathological change occurs.

Answer A defect in organic binding of thyroid iodine.

Question Can Hashimoto's disease present with signs of hyperthyroidism.

Answer Yes. In about one-fifth of the patients mild thyrotoxicosis occurs in the early stages of the disease.

Question Does hypothyroidism finally develop.

Answer Yes. Even in patients who are euthyroid when first seen overt myxoedema eventually occurs, often after several years.

Question What laboratory tests confirm the diagnosis of Hashimoto's disease.

Answer Tests designed to establish the presence of antibodies to:

1 Thyroglobulin.

2 Microsomal antigen.

3 Second colloid antigen.

4 Cell surface antigen.

5 Thyroxine and tri-iodothyronine.

Comment In this patient the presence of thyroid microsomal antigens was estimated by complement fixation. The titre was high.

Question In the normal population can microsomal antibodies be identified.

Answer Yes, in very low titre in about seven per cent of the population.

Question What is the most sensitive test for hypothyroidism.

Answer The circulating level of TSH. Reduction of thyroid function, automatically, by means of the normal 'feedback' mechanism, raises the level of circulating TSH.

Question What is the treatment of Hashimoto's disease.

Answer Fine needle aspiration or open biopsy in order to exclude malignant disease or the presence of a lymphoma followed by the administration of L-thyroxine, 0.1 mg bd or tds.

Question What is the action of L-thyroxine.

Answer

1 It prevents the overt symptoms of myxoedema developing.

2 The suggestion has been made that by reducing the circulating level of TSH it so alters the characteristics of the thyrocytes that the autoimmune signal decreases.

3 It eventually reduces the size of the goitre.

Question What are the common symptoms of myxoedema.

Answer

1 Undue tiredness.

2 Weakness.

3 Lethargy.

4 Increased sensitivity to cold.

5 Hoarseness of the voice due to thickening of the cords.

6 Increasing weight.

7 Loss of hair from the scalp and outer third of the eyebrows.

8 Increasing coarseness of the skin, particularly noted in the face.

Question What are the chief signs of myxoedema.

Answer

1 A swollen waxy face due to the deposition of mucin in the connective and subcutaneous tissues.

2 Pale, dry skin.

3 Stiffness of the muscles.

4 A carpal tunnel syndrome.

5 Rarely signs of cerebellar degeneration resulting in dysarthria, ataxia, an intention tremor.

6 Very rarely an organic psychosis, 'myxoedema madness'.

7 Signs of heart failure due to enlargement of the heart and tamponade from a pericardial effusion.

Comment In this patient, despite the presence of a goitre and marked immunological evidence of autoimmune thyroiditis the patient had neither symptoms nor signs of incipient myxoedema.

Physical examination There were no physical signs present in any system, but examination of the abdomen revealed a huge mass approximately the size of a water melon descending from beneath the left costal margin. The mass appeared to be solid but its outline was smooth. No notch was present on its anterior border to suggest that it was the spleen and pressure in the left loin did not increase the prominence or the definition of the swelling. It was dull to percussion and, therefore, thought to be solid and it moved downwards on inspiration.

Question What possibilities suggest themselves.

Answer The most obvious, and that accepted by the majority of surgeons who examined this patient, was that the swelling represented a large solid swelling arising on the left lobe of the liver. However, to postulate that the swelling represented a primary liver tumour or a secondary tumour appeared out of the question in view of the two year history and the absence of any deterioration in the patient's general condition.

Question What types of primary malignant tumours occur in the liver.

Answer

1 Primary hepatoma, the incidence of this tumour is related in white races to that of alcoholic cirrhosis. However, in the African Bantu primary liver cancer is the commonest form of malignant disease found in this ethnic group. The cause for this may be both environmental and dietary. Other than cirrhosis the incidence of primary hepatoma is high in haemochromatosis and patients in whom a chronic active hepatitis is caused by the hepatitis B virus.

2 Cholangiocarcinoma, bile duct carcinoma. The tumours grow slowly and spreading directly along the bile ducts cause painless progressive jaundice.

3 Hepatoblastoma, this tumour belongs to the class of embryonal tumours. It is rare and most commonly appears in the first few years of life.

4 Angiosarcoma, this rare tumour may occur either in the infant or the adult. In the adult it may be associated with exposure to vinylchloride monomer which is used in industry to form the common, non-carcinogenic, plastic polyvinyl chloride by polymerization.

5 Fibrolamellar carcinoma.

Comment Since primary tumours of the liver are rare and as previously stated the history in this patient extended over two years this diagnosis seemed highly inappropriate. Furthermore, to postulate metastatic growth seemed wholly unreasonable in view of the length of the history and the absence of systemic symptoms.

Question Are there any benign tumours which might account for the physical findings.

Answer

1 Hepatic adenoma. These tumours may reach considerable size and furthermore, can produce episodic pain due to degeneration and haemorrhage within the tumour.

2 Harmatoma, this tumour-like malformation of normal tissues in disorderly arrangement usually presents in childhood but may cause abdominal enlargement and vomiting.

Comment In scraping the barrel for some other acceptable diagnosis the suggestion was put forward that this tumour could be a giant benign leiomyoma arising from the greater curvature of the stomach. However, this type of tumour normally presents with the symptoms of anaemia due to chronic blood loss or causes a massive haematemesis due to ulceration of the mucosa over the surface of the tumour. Grate and others examined the presentation of benign gastric neoplasms and found that symptoms were rarely present in tumours less than 3 cm in diameter and that the majority of those larger than 6 cm had all produced symptoms.

Question What investigation would you request.

Answer Ultrasound examination in the belief that this would, at least, localize the position of the tumour.

It showed gross distension of the abdomen corresponding to the site of the mass with gross thickening of the wall of the stomach in its distal portion. A diagnosis of gastric outflow obstruction was made. At the same time as the ultrasound examination was performed a plain X-ray of the chest was also performed. This is shown in Fig. 4.1.

Question What does this show.

Answer A fluid level suggesting the presence of an incarcerated, i.e. irreducible hiatus hernia.

Comment Following these investigations a nasogastric tube was passed and 5 litres of fluid were rapidly aspirated with the result that the abdominal tumour completely disappeared.

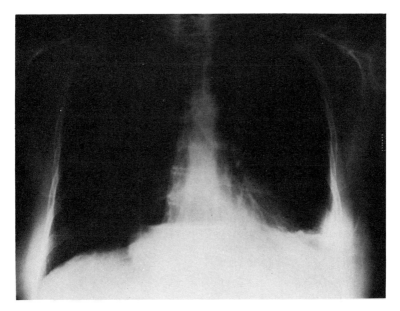

4.1

Question What conclusion would you draw from this.

Answer The only reasonable explanation is that we are dealing not only with a para-oesophageal hernia but also with a volvulus of the stomach.

Question How could this diagnosis be established.

Answer By barium meal, the result of which is shown in Figs 4.2(a) and (b).

Comment This patient was also endoscoped. The instrument was passed with ease and the following comments made by the observer. Gastric erosions were present high in the lesser curvature, the instrument retroflexed on its own to show a view of the scope in the cardia, a deep ridge, and the pyloric opening next to it. No bile was seen in the stomach. High on the greater curve was a gastric ulcer.

Question What symptoms normally occur in the presence of an uncomplicated para-oesophageal hernia.

Answer The two commonest symptoms are epigastric fullness and intermittent vomiting.

Question One of the chief symptoms in the patient under discussion was severe abdominal pain; what does this imply.

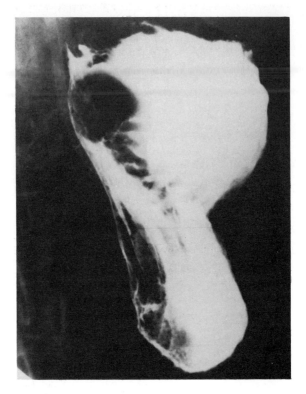

4.2a

Answer The presence of incarceration and obstruction.

Question What complications occur in association with a para-oesophageal hernia.

Answer

1 Incarceration, i.e. irreducibility, this is certainly present in this patient since the presence of a fluid level indicates irreducibility.

2 Obstruction.

3 Gangrene.

4 Perforation.

5 Ulceration, this nearly always occurs where the greater curve abuts against the hiatus.

6 In the presence of ulceration, a severe haematemesis.

7 Volvulus.

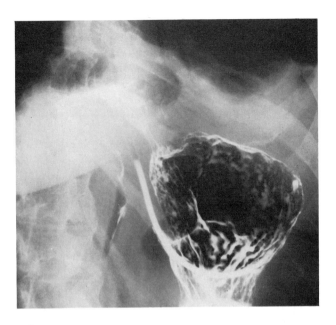

4.2b

Question What types of gastric volvulus occur.

Answer Volvulus of the stomach is classified according to the plane around which rotation occurs.

1 Organo-axial: the plane of rotation occurs around an axis running from the cardio-oesophageal junction to the pyloric canal.

2 Axial rotation: this occurs around a vertical axis through the cardio-oesophageal junction.

Question Which is the commoner type.

Answer The organo-axial. Consequent upon this rotation the pylorus and pyloric antrum are directed downwards as is shown in Fig. 4.2(b). This condition must be distinguished from the 'cup and spill' cascade stomach.

Question How common is a gastric volvulus in the presence of a para-oesophageal hernia.

Answer In the largest series reported organo-axial rotation occurred in 20 per cent of patients.

Question What is the anatomical difference between a para-oesophageal hernia and a parahiatal hernia.

Answer In a true parahiatal hernia a component of the diaphragm is present between the herniated stomach and the oesophagus.

Question What is the anatomical disposition of the cardia and fundus of the stomach in an uncomplicated para-oesophageal hernia.

Answer The oesophago-gastric junction remains posterior to the sac into which the fundus herniates, being held in position by the intact phreno-oesophageal ligament. The hiatal deficit is always anterior to the oesophagus and as the hernia enlarges so organo-axial rotation tends to occur with the greater curve moving in the direction of the right shoulder.

Comment In this patient the acute symptoms with which the patient presented were rapidly relieved by the passage of a nasogastric tube. However, in some patients this treatment is ineffective since the tube never reaches the gastric sump which was at first thought in this patient to represent a tumour.

When relief cannot be achieved by the passage of a nasogastric tube immediate surgery is required.

Question What are the chief steps in the surgical treatment of this patient.
Answer
    1 Open the abdomen through a midline or left paramedian incision.
    2 Reduce the hernia, there are never any adhesions between the stomach and the sac.

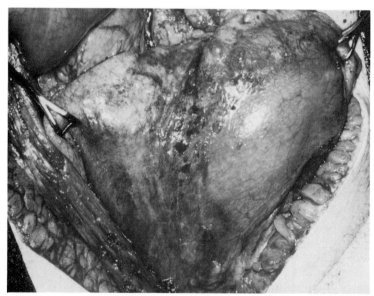

4.3

3 Remove the sac from the posterior mediastinum and excise it.

4 Repair the hiatal defect.

Hill suggests that the hiatus is repaired posterior to the oesophagus and that following this repair the stomach is fixed to the posterior surface of the anterior abdominal wall by creating a temporary gastrostomy. In this case the crura were approximated anterior to the oesophagus and a gastrostomy was not performed. The argument in favour of a gastrostomy is the incidence of recurrent volvulus even following reduction of the hernia and repair of the hiatus.

Question Should para-oesophageal hernias be repaired in the absence of severe symptoms.

Answer A review of the literature on this subject suggests that reduction and repair should be performed following diagnosis because the operative mortality in an uncomplicated case is low whereas the mortality following strangulation is high.

Comment This patient was seen six months after reduction and repair of the hiatus and was symptom-free. Figure 4.3 shows the stomach with the ulcerating constriction running across the serosal surface as found at operation in this patient.

5

A Caucasian male, 62 years of age, was admitted complaining of severe epigastric pain of approximately nine years duration, worse in the last six weeks. Recently the pain had been associated with severe constant backache in the lower thoracic region. These attacks occurred at any time of the day and night and were frequently disturbing his sleep. The pain was relieved by vomiting. His bowels were regular. Examination revealed only tenderness in the epigastric region.

Previous history Two years prior to admission he had been investigated for a complaint of dyspepsia, 'wind' and lower abdominal colic. The last symptom occurred some two to three times a day and was only relieved by passing flatus which was normally followed by a loose motion. At that time a sigmoidoscopy and barium enema had been performed both revealing no abnormality. However, a barium meal had revealed a gastric ulcer.

Question What features found on the barium meal suggest that the ulcer is benign.

Answer

1   The ulcer crater projects beyond the wall of the stomach to appear as a smooth pit whose borders are rounded.

2   When repeated healing and breakdown of the ulcer has occurred leading to submucosal fibrosis the rugal folds radiate inwards towards the crater (Fig. 5.1).

Question What further investigation is required.

Answer Endoscopy. It is essential in a man of 62 years of age to have histological proof that the gastric ulcer is benign particularly in view of the increasingly severe symptoms. Endoscopy using a flexible instrument allows the operator not only to see the ulcer but also to take brushing from the edge of the ulcer or multiple biopsies from its edges. In this case the ulcer was found to be benign.

Question What errors may follow endoscopic biopsy.

Answer

1   As in the case of biliary gastritis the diagnosis of malignancy may be missed.

2   The pathologist may mistake small elements of regenerating epithelium at the edge of the ulcer which have grown down into the submucosa as evidence of malignancy.

Question What endoscopic appearances distinguish a benign from a gastric ulcer.

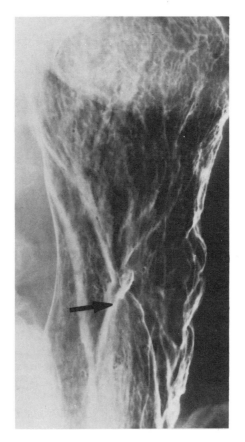

5.1

Answer A benign ulcer should have clear-cut overhanging edges with no thickening of the adjacent mucosa although this will appear oedematous.

Question What are the chief pathological features of a chronic gastric ulcer.

Answer

1 The ulcer is round or oval lying across the lesser curve, usually somewhat higher in the female than the male because of the proximal extension of the antral mucosa in the former, particularly with advancing age.

2 The edges are clear cut but tend to overhang the ulcer to produce a flask shaped defect.

3 The base of the ulcer has four recognizable layers, from the floor downwards.

(a) A narrow zone of fibrino-purulent exudate.

(b) A layer of acidophilic necrotic tissue.

(c) A zone of granulation tissue.

(d) An outer layer of dense scar tissue in which lymphoid aggregates are present, the smaller arteries show evidence of thrombo-endarteritis obliterans.

Question In which part of the stomach do benign ulcers most commonly occur.

Answer At the incisura angularis on the lesser curve. However, whilst this is the most common site, over 50 per cent occurring in this anatomical position, an important factor determining the site of the ulcer on the lesser curve is the variable distribution of the antral mucosa since the majority of gastric ulcers develop at the junction of the body and antral mucosa.

Question What diameter can chronic gastric ulcers reach.

Answer Gastric ulcers are most frequently 2 cm or less in diameter, the crater lying across the lesser curve in a saddle shaped form. Occasionally, in older women especially, a gastric ulcer can be extremely large extending over several centimetres reaching from the incisura to the cardia.

Question What is the incidence of chronic gastric ulceration.

Answer Post-mortem studies suggest the incidence of active ulceration in men is somewhat less than three per cent and in women somewhat greater than one per cent.

Question What is the incidence of malignancy degeneration in benign gastric ulceration (ulcer-cancer).

Answer Although previously thought to be as high as 30 per cent this figure has now been reduced to seven per cent.

Question What pathological criteria establish the diagnoses of ulcer cancer.

Answer

1 There must be definite evidence of a pre-existing ulcer showing all the pathological features described in the answer to the fourth question.

2 There must be definite evidence of malignant change at the edge of the ulcer quite distinct from any attempt at epithelial regeneration.

3 In a true ulcer-cancer the base is never invaded.

Comment Many authorities classify gastric ulcers in the following manner:

Type I. Ulcers developing in the prepyloric zone. These have more in common with duodenal than gastric ulcers since they are associated with a high acid output.

Type II. Gastric ulcers associated with duodenal ulceration. First a duodenal ulcer develops, the patient being a hypersecretor, following which a gastric ulcer develops as a complication of pyloric obstruction. This type is said to account for approximately 14 per cent of all gastric ulcers.

Type III. This is the commonest type of gastric ulcer and is always associated with marked hyposecretion which suggests that they are caused by a deficiency in mucus production.

Under normal circumstances acid penetrates gastric mucus at 1 mm/h and in a normal stomach an increase in acid secretion is accompanied by an increase in mucus production in order to protect the mucosa. Two hypotheses have been advanced to explain how this natural barrier may break down.

1 Since no cell can continue to secrete indefinitely without rest a prolonged period of acid oversecretion might overwhelm the mucus secreting cells. This would be particularly applicable to Type II gastric ulcers.

2 Lack of mucus secretion may be caused by relative anoxia of the mucus secreting cells.

Question What role, if any, do the prostaglandins play in the development of a peptic ulcer.

Answer Experimental studies indicate that the prostaglandins can prevent disruption of the mucosal barrier by agents such as bile salts, aspirin and alcohol. Other studies also indicate that the prostaglandins can stimulate mucus production possibly by increasing mucosal perfusion since these chemicals are powerful gastric capillary dilators.

Other possible mechanisms by which endogenous and exogenous prostaglandins may exert a protective action are by:

1 Stimulating (HCO_3^-) secretions.

2 Maintaining normal ionic flux across the mucosa.

3 Enhancing mucosal repair and cell replication.

4 Inhibiting acid secretion.

Question Is it possible to explain the large bowel symptoms exhibited by this patient.

Answer Two alternative explanations are possible:

1 that coincidentally the patient suffered from the 'irritable bowel' syndrome.

2 the symptoms may have been due to the adverse effects of magnesium trisilicate with which the patient had been treated for many years. Ninety-five per cent of magnesium trisilicate, dosage normally

between 0.5–2 g, is retained within the gastro-intestinal tract only five per cent being absorbed. Retained within the gastro-intestinal tract it acts as a saline laxative.

Question What might explain the recent onset of back pain.

Answer Uncomplicated gastric ulcers are frequently associated with pain in the interscapular region but the recent onset of the symptom suggests that the ulcer crater has penetrated the pancreas, a hypothesis supported by the onset of severe pain at night.

Question What treatment regime would you prescribe.

Answer Ranitidine 150 mg twice daily for a period of six months together with carbenoxolone sodium 100 mg three times a day for one week followed by 50 mg three times a day. The action of ranitidine is described on p. 68. Carbenoxolone has a marked anti-inflammatory action which appears to act locally on the stomach stimulating the production of protective mucus.

Question Has carbenoxolone any adverse side effects.

Answer Carbenoxolone sodium may produce sodium and water retention leading to oedema, alkalosis, hypertension, hypokalaemia. These effects are particularly liable to occur in the elderly. The symptomatic presentation of these various side effects include headache, oedema, breathlessness, cardiac failure and if hypokalaemia develops muscular weakness. In this patient there is no contraindication to its use since there is no history of cardiovascular disease.

Question What other drugs have been shown to be effective in the treatment of chronic gastric ulceration.

Answer Colloidal bismuth subcitrate, tripotassium dicitrato-bismuthate, a complex bismuth salt of citric acid and sucralfate.

Question What is the action of colloidal bismuth subcitrate.

Answer At an acid pH, colloidal bismuth selectively chelates with the proteinaceous material in the base of an ulcer forming a protective coating thus preventing the destructive action of acid, pepsin and bile. In addition this drug also inhibits the activity of pepsin. In terms of healing rates this drug is roughly equivalent to cimetidine.

Question What, if any, are the side effects of this drug.

Answer Darkening of the tongue, teeth and stools. In addition, the liquid preparation has an unpleasant ammonical taste and smell. This drug is not at present recommended for maintenance therapy.

Question What is the action of sucralfate.

Answer This drug has a similar action to colloidal bismuth. In the stomach in the presence of an acidic environment, polymerization leads to the formation of a viscous paste-like substance which selectively binds to the proteinaceous material in the base of the ulcer producing a protective layer against the further action of acid, pepsin and bile.

In addition this drug also selectively binds acid. Endoscopically controlled trials have shown that 1 g qds is as effective as an H_2 antagonist. There are no side effects since the drug is not absorbed.

Comment This patient was treated in the manner described without relief and a decision to operate was made only after two years.

Question What operations have been described for the treatment of gastric ulceration.

Answer

1 For many years the 'standard' operation for the treatment of a chronic, intractable, gastric ulcer situated in the region of the incisura, i.e. the Type III ulcer has been a Bilroth I type of gastric resection. In this operation the ulcer, together with a portion of the body and the whole of the antrum, is removed. The lesser curve is reconstituted and a gastro-duodenal anastomosis performed. The side effects of this operation are similar to those following the classic Polya type of gastrectomy since in both the pyloric sphincter is resected.

Approximately 75 per cent of patients obtain a highly satisfactory result as measured by Visick's classification. The remainder suffer in varying degree from the various post-gastrectomy syndromes and in most series recurrent ulceration is reported in about five per cent.

2 Recently papers have appeared in the literature suggesting that both Type II and III ulcers could be better treated by either a truncal vagotomy and pyloroplasty or by highly selective vagotomy together with excision of the ulcer.

However, a search of the surgical literature does not appear to substantiate these suggestions. Various reports make it clear that truncal vagotomy and pyloroplasty produces no clear cut benefit over the classical Bilroth operation. In addition, in 1979, Duthie and his collaborators compared the results of HSV and excision of the ulcer with Bilroth resection in the treatment of Type III ulcers. They found in their randomized series no advantage of HSV over the Bilroth resection and in addition found the recurrent ulcer rate to be 15 per cent after HSV even having excised the original ulcer as compared to seven per cent for Bilroth I gastrectomy.

Question What specific anatomical complication is responsible for the majority of deaths following a Bilroth I gastrectomy.

Answer Leakage from the point at which the reconstituted lesser curve is anastomized to the duodenum.

Question What is the Visick Classification.

Answer Visick was a York surgeon who classified his post-gastrectomy results in the following manner.

Grade I. No gastric symptoms.

Grade II. Mild symptoms easily controlled by adjustment of diet or way of life.

Grade III. Mild symptoms *not* controllable but not interfering with way of life.

Grade IV. Symptoms worse than before operation, patient incapacitated.

Comment Laparotomy revealed an ulcer 2 cm in diameter extending distally from the incisura angularis. No adherence and, therefore, no penetration of the pancreas was found. A Bilroth I operation was performed, no deformity of the duodenum being present. Recovery was uninterrupted and the patient returned home on the 14th postoperative day.

6

A Caucasian male aged 57 years was admitted complaining of intermittent upper abdominable pain after meals and also at night for several months. He described the pain as gnawing in character. Although the pain appeared to be particularly severe late in the evening it had not interfered with sleep. The patient had lost 5 kilos over six months.

Previous medical history Twenty years previously he had undergone a truncal vagotomy and posterior no-loop retrocolic gastroenterostomy for the treatment of an intractable duodenal ulcer.

Physical examination Inspection. This revealed a thin somewhat emaciated male.

Cerebrovascular system	No abnormality detected.
Respiratory system	Evidence of chronic bronchitis, restricted air entry and scattered rhonci.
Abdominal examination	A left upper paramedian incision was present.
Palpation	Diffuse tenderness was present in the upper abdomen. PR negative.

Question What three conditions might be the cause of these symptoms.
Answer
1   Recurrent ulceration, either duodenal or anastomotic.
2   Bile reflux gastritis.
3   Carcinoma of the stomach.

Question Where do recurrent ulcers develop following a truncal vagotomy and gastroenterostomy.
Answer Recurrent ulceration occurs in the duodenum or alternatively an anastomotic ulcer develops in the efferent loop immediately adjacent to the stoma.

Question What is the incidence of recurrent ulcer following truncal vagotomy and gastroenterostomy.
Answer The majority of published British Series report the incidence of recurrent ulceration as being between four and 12 per cent. A somewhat higher figure has been reported in the United States, e.g. 13 per cent by Walters and Mobley of the Mayo Clinic and 24 per cent by Nobles of Memphis.

Question What determines the incidence of recurrent ulceration.
Answer The 'completeness' or otherwise of the vagotomy.

Question What is the principle effect of vagotomy.

Answer Truncal vagotomy reduces the basal acid output and peak acid output in response to stimulation by histamine, pentagastrin or meat extracts by 60–80 per cent and 50–70 per cent respectively. For further discussion see Viva 8.

Comment In this patient a barium meal revealed a superficial gastric ulcer proximal to the anastomosis. Endoscopy was performed; biopsy material showed the characteristic changes of chronic atrophic gastritis and bile reflux gastritis. He commenced ranitidine.

Question What is the incidence of bile reflux gastritis following gastric surgery.

Answer Savage (1979) surveyed a series of 63 patients by means of endoscopy and multiple mucosal biopsies who had been subjected to gastric surgery. These patients were part of a larger series of 224 patients all of whom had been operated upon by a single surgeon. At the time of the survey 115 patients were still alive and 63 patients agreed to be investigated. The time interval between operation and endoscopy varied between 15 and 27 years. His principle finding was that the gastric mucosa was histologically abnormal in all the patients investigated although none of the 63 patients had had sufficiently severe symptoms to warrant seeking advice from their own doctor, the majority being completely asymptomatic.

It is, however, recognized that bile reflux gastritis can be a cause of upper abdominal pain although there is little correlation between the severity of the symptoms and the histological changes in the mucosa. It is also recognized that the condition may progress to dysplasia and, therefore, may be potentially malignant.

Question What is the incidence of cancer in the gastric remnant following gastrectomy.

Answer All reports confirm an increased incidence of gastric cancer following gastric surgery particularly after gastrectomy but the frequency in different series is variously recorded as between one and two per cent.

Question Does the type of gastrectomy affect the incidence.

Answer Bilroth I gastrectomy is followed by fewer gastric cancers than the Bilroth II (Polya).

Question What is the time interval between operation and the development of gastric cancer.

Answer The incidence of malignancy is variously reported as reaching a maximum some 15–30 years following surgery.

Question What are the principle symptoms associated with gastric remnant cancer.

Answer Abdominal pain, weight loss and anorexia.

Question What are the principle symptoms associated with reflux biliary gastritis.

Answer Persistent epigastric pain and nausea, unrelieved by antacids and worse after eating. Bilious vomiting may occur particularly early in the morning or following meals. Weight loss is common. In a small number of patients as illustrated by this patient the symptoms associated with reflux may develop several years after surgery.

Question How would you differentiate cancer in the gastric remnant from reflux biliary gastritis.

Answer The most important investigation is endoscopy since any lesion observed can then be biopsied.

Comment In this patient a succession of endoscopies were performed, usually following the failure of one particular form of medical treatment to relieve the symptoms. These various biopsies, taken at intervals over a period of several months, showed evidence of marked biliary gastritis with extensive intestinal metaplasia.

Question What is the incidence of symptomatic biliary reflux.

Answer It is variously reported as between five and 35 per cent.

Question What is the cause of the mucosal changes in this condition.

Answer It is now considered that the bile acids and salts exert a detergent effect on the gastric mucosa. However, in a symptomatic patient the infusion of bile alone produces less severe symptoms in fewer patients than does the infusion of autologous intestinal contents.

Question What are the histological changes associated with biliary reflux gastritis.

Answer Morson classified the changes as follows:

1   Chronic superficial gastritis.

2   Atrophic gastritis.

3   Gastric atrophy.

Both chronic superficial gastritis and atrophic gastritis may be quiescent or active and the changes associated with atrophic gastritis may remain stationary for many years.

Question What are the chief histological features of active superficial gastritis.

Answer

1   The mucosa is oedematous and shows features of vascular congestion.

2   The epithelium shows degenerative and regenerative changes. The cells are more cuboidal than columnar. The lamina propria contains polymorphonuclear leucocytes, lymphocytes and plasma

cells. When active, numerous polymorphonuclear leucocytes are present which disappear as the disease becomes quiescent.

Question What are the chief histological changes in chronic atrophic gastritis.

Answer
1 A reduction in the number of chief and parietal cells in the mucosa of the body and fundus of the stomach.
2 Atrophy of the glands in the deep zone of the antral mucosa.
3 Metaplasia towards an intestinal type of epithelium.

Question What are the chief features of intestinal metaplasia in the gastric mucosa.

Answer The most characteristic features are the presence of goblet cells of intestinal type together with columnar cells. The latter have a prominent striated border of microvilli. Paneth cells, absent from normal gastric mucosa, are also found in large numbers.

Comment Chronic atrophic gastritis has recently been classified into two types:

Type A. In this type anti-parietal cell antibodies are found. The condition spares the antrum, affecting chiefly the body and fundus of the stomach leading to hypo or achlorhydria and impaired Vitamin B_{12} absorption.

Type B. In which antibodies are not found. Vitamin B_{12} absorption is not affected, acid secretion remains normal and in which the changes begin distally and spread slowly proximally. This is the type associated with bile reflux, uraemia, cirrhosis and campylobacter.

Question Is intestinal metaplasia in the stomach a premalignant condition.

Answer Yes. The evidence for this is as follows:
1 The incidence of intestinal metaplasia is significantly greater in the presence of a gastric cancer.
2 In early cancers of the stomach a transition between metaplasia and early gastric cancer can be frequently seen.
3 The distribution of intestinal metaplasia is similar to the distribution of primary carcinoma of the stomach.
4 Approximately 50 per cent of all invasive cancers of the stomach are of the intestinal cell type.

Question What medical regimes have been suggested to relieve symptomatic biliary gastritis.

Answer
1 A low fat diet in an attempt to decrease biliary secretion.
2 Avoidance of alcohol and smoking.

3 The administration of metoclopramide to increase the rate of gastric emptying.

Question What is the chief pharmacological action of metoclopramide.

Answer This drug has central and anti-emetic properties and a positive effect on intestinal motility. Gastric peristalsis is increased leading to an increase in the gastric emptying rate.

Comment All these various medical regimes were administered to this patient with little symptomatic relief.

It was, therefore, decided to take down the gastroenterostomy and return intestinal continuity to normal. This was performed and no evidence of recurrent duodenal or anastomotic ulceration was found. The patient developed a relatively severe chest infection which responded to physiotherapy and antibiotics and thereafter all appeared to be well. On the fourth post-operative day the nasogastric tube was removed and the patient passed some flatus.

However, on the following evening the patient began to vomit although within 48 hours he again settled. A gastrografin was performed; this showed some delay in gastric emptying and in the region of the antrum some thickened folds of mucosa were seen which were interpreted by the radiologist as being due to the recent surgery.

In view of the delayed emptying the gastric emptying time was measured before and after the administration of the drug Cisapride 10 mg. This demonstrated marked delay before the administration of the drug and relatively normal emptying following its administration.

However, 48 hours later the patient again vomited large volumes of gastric contents.

Question Why should the patient vomit.

Answer This patient had been previously subjected to a truncal vagotomy which is normally followed by gross changes in gastric motility. Even many years later electromyographic studies show residual changes in antral motility.

Question Who introduced truncal vagotomy as a method of treating duodenal ulceration.

Answer Dragstedt in 1943, whose inspiration came from experimental work performed by Hartzell in 1929 in the dog who showed that division of the vagi in this animal decreased gastric acidity. The truncal vagotomies by Dragstedt were performed via thoracotomy incisions but it was very soon recognized that truncal vagotomy alone was followed in a high proportion of patients by gastric atony.

In 1948 Moore found, for example, that whereas in normal individuals barium left the stomach in 30–90 seconds in patients in whom a truncal vagotomy had been performed, the emptying time might extend to between 20 and 140 minutes. Thus the original operation was first abandoned and later revived performing the truncal vagotomy via the abdomen and at the same time performing either a pyloroplasty, antrectomy or gastroenterostomy. However, many observers noted that even without drainage gastric motility and gastric emptying improved with the passage of time and indeed on the basis of this evidence McMahon and others in 1978 treated nine patients who were complaining of persistent abdominal pain and intermittent vomiting following truncal vagotomy and gastroenterostomy by merely taking down the gastroenterostomy and restoring gastro-intestinal continuity. All these nine patients did well, none developed gastric retention and all were symptomatically improved.

Question What alternative surgical procedure has been suggested to relieve reflux biliary gastritis.

Answer Perform an antrectomy, anastomose the gastric remnant to a Roux loop and anastomose the afferent loop at least 40 cm distal to the stomach so that the reflux of bile and pancreatic secretions into the stomach is diminished. When bile vomiting follows a standard Bilroth II, Polya type gastrectomy this operation must be accompanied by a vagotomy to avoid the possible danger of an anastomotic ulcer developing.

Question Do these anti-reflux operations result in reversal of the histological changes in the antral mucosa.

Answer Yes. Nearly all reports which compare the histological changes present in pre-operative and post-operative biopsy specimens show that considerable histological improvement occurs following anti-reflux procedures. Furthermore, functional tests show that achlorhydria and hypochlorhydria may revert to normosecretion after surgery.

Comment This patient continued to vomit despite a barium meal showing no hold up and after a period of some three weeks during which the patient was maintained by intravenous parenteral nutrition, a decision was made to re-operate upon him.

At operation a formal Bilroth II, Polya type gastrectomy was performed. The specimen was opened at the time of the operation to reveal an invasive gastric cancer. Fortunately, none of the six lymph nodes removed appeared to be involved in malignant disease and the patient made an uninterrupted recovery.

Question What are the most important late complications of a Bilroth II Polya type gastrectomy.

Answer

1 Dumping.
2 Malabsorption.
3 Metabolic bone disease.
4 Reactive hypoglycaemia.
5 Cancer of the gastric remnant.

Comment In only one of the many biopsies taken from this patient was there any suggestion of possible malignant change and a further biopsy taken from approximately the same area was said to be normal. Unfortunately, at the time of 'unpicking' the gastroenterostomy external inspection and both external and internal palpation of the pyloric antrum revealed no abnormality.

This case emphasizes two major points.

1 It is unwise to rely too heavily on endoscopy, particularly in a stomach already the site of an operation.

Two major technical difficulties are associated with endoscopy in this type of stomach. First, the stomach is difficult to inflate and secondly, it is difficult to obtain biopsy specimens from previous sites with any degree of certainty.

2 How the result of one investigation can impair surgical judgement.

7

A 72-year-old white male was admitted complaining of painless constipation of four weeks duration. Over the period he had passed no
blood and had had no intervening attacks of diarrhoea. His appetite
had been poor for approximately six weeks and he had developed
a bad taste in the mouth and also occasional vomiting. He had lost
14 kilograms in weight in eight weeks.

Previous medical history Thirty years previously he had undergone a
bilateral pyelolithotomy for renal calculi. Three years previously he
had suffered a myocardial infarct; he complained of angina which
was relieved by nitrites.

Two years previously he had developed mild haematuria, nocturia,
difficulty and frequency of micturition, together with pain in the left
loin. Examination on admission revealed bilateral lumbar herniae,
the whole length of both lumbar wounds having broken down to
produce massive uncontrollable incisional herniae. Rectal examination revealed a moderate enlargement of the prostate.

Question What investigations would you have ordered to elucidate
the cause of his urinary symptoms two years prior to his present
admission.

Answer

1   Urine microscopy to identify either red cells, malignant cells or
both.

2   Plasma electrolytes to exclude renal failure and hypercalaemia.

3   Bacteriological examination of the urine.

4   Urine flow rate.

5   An intravenous pyelogram.

6   ECG to assess the cardiac condition.

The results were as follows:

1   Urine microscopy showed red cells but no malignant cells.

2   The plasma electrolyte levels were within normal limits.

3   No significant bacterial growth was found in the urine.

4   The flow rate was reduced, 8 ml/second.

5   The plain X-ray of the abdomen showed a solitary calculus in
the left renal area and multiple scattered areas of calcification in the
right kidney. The intravenous pyelogram shows that on neither side
is there any obstruction. Pre- and post-evacuation films of the bladder
showed significant retention of urine with evidence of trabeculation.

Question What is the probable chemical composition of these calculi.

Answer These stones are probably composed of calcium oxalate and/or phosphate. In any published series this is the most common type of kidney stone. Much less common are stones composed of calcium phosphate plus magnesium ammonium phosphate which are associated with infection. Rarer still are the metabolic stones composed of uric acid, xanthine or cystine, the last being the rarest type of stone.

Question What conditions are associated with calcium oxalate and/or phosphate stones.

Answer The great majority, i.e. approximately 80 per cent of calcium stone formers are associated with idiopathic hypercalciuria, i.e. they excrete larger than normal amounts of calcium for which no explanation can be found. However, similar stones develop in conditions which predispose to a high level of calcium excretion, e.g. primary hyperparathyroidism, vitamin D intoxication, sarcoidosis and patients in whom osseous metastases are present. Specific causes of a high oxalate excretion include primary (hereditary) hyperoxaluria and enteric hyperoxaluria.

Question What conditions are associated with calcium phosphate/ magnesium ammonium phosphate stones.

Answer Infection of the urinary tract by urea-splitting organisms.

Question What are the common urea splitting organisms found in the urine.

Answer *Proteus, Escherichia coli, Klebsiella, Pseudomonas aeruginosa.*

Question What factors predispose to the development of a urinary tract infection.

Answer The commonest cause is an organic or functional obstruction to the free drainage of urine. Examples of the former include prostatism, examples of the latter include vesico-ureteric reflux and neurogenic bladder.

Question What is the mechanism by which urea-splitting organisms cause stone production.

Answer The urea splitting organisms secrete urease which splits urea into carbon dioxide and urea. This leads to a high urinary pH so that calcium phosphate is precipitated and in addition the high ammonia concentration in an alkaline urine causes the precipitation of triple phosphate. Other factors may also be operating including the metabolism of urinary citrate which is normally one of the mechanisms by which the solubility of calcium salts in the urine is maintained.

Question What factor other than the supersaturation of the urine with calcium oxalate and phosphate is required to cause calcium stone formation.

Answer A diminution in the urinary concentration of compounds which inhibit the crystallization of these salts. The level of inhibitory activity in the urine depends upon the relative concentrations of glycosaminoglycans and urates. The former are potent inhibitors but this inhibitory activity is reduced in the presence of high concentrations of uric acid.

Question What is the macroscopic appearance of a calcium oxalate stone

Answer The typical calcium oxalate stone is small, spikey and frequently brown due to being covered with altered blood.

Question What factors, other than some specific metabolic abnormality such as primary hyperparathyroid suggest that a patient will develop recurrent stones as in this individual.

Answer

1 A high urinary calcium concentration.

2 A higher than normal oxalate concentration in the urine.

3 The presence of a large number of calcium oxalate crystals in the urine.

Question What dietary advice would you give to help avoid recurrent calcium oxalate/phosphate stone formation.

Answer

1 Increase fluid intake in order to reduce the risk of precipitating solutes. This is not so easily achieved because the estimated urine volume required to achieve adequate dilution over the whole 24 hour period is 3 litres.

2 Avoidance of calcium and oxalate rich foods. Prominent among the former are milk and cheese and among the latter rhubarb, strawberries and spinach.

Question What drugs can be used to control hypercalciuria.

Answer The thiazide diuretics, e.g. chlorothiazide sodium (Saluric, Merck, Sharpe and Dohme).

The administration of this drug lowers the urinary calcium concentration and also the degree of crystalluria.

Another drug which affects the urinary calcium is cellulose phosphate which, if taken just after meals, combines with calcium in the gastrointestinal tract so preventing the absorption of dietary calcium.

Question What are the chief modes of presentation of renal calculi.

Answer

1 Pain. The pain is of two types, a small stone which is mobile within a calix or within the renal pelvis may give rise to classical renal colic whereas a large immobile calculus may be asymptomatic or cause a constant dull loin pain.

2 Haematuria. This may be either microscopic or very obvious.

3 Urinary tract infection, this may be acute if combined with obstruction when there develops severe loin pain, pyrexia and tachycardia.

Comment This patient was originally treated by bilateral pyelolithotomy. In recent years, however, open surgery is being replaced by two other methods, i.e.

1 Percutaneous surgery in which the offending stone is either removed mechanically or shattered by ultrasonic waves or electro-hydraulic probes.

2 Extracorporeal shock wave lithotripsy. In this technique the shock waves generated by an ultrashort high tension underwater electrical discharge are accurately focused on the calculus; a success rate of 92 per cent has been claimed for this method by the London Litho-tripter Centre. The sole disadvantage of this technique is the high initial cost of the equipment in a field in which improving technology may soon make present day machines obsolete.

Question What treatment would you advise for his difficulty in micturition.

Answer Transurethral prostatectomy. This was performed, 20 g of benign prostatic tissue being removed. A Foley catheter with closed drainage was left *in situ* for three days. He was discharged home on the fourth post-operative day.

Question What part of the prostate is involved in benign hyperplasia.

Answer The central group of glands which in older men enlarge at the expense of the peripheral glandular tissue.

Question What may be the cause of the phenomenon.

Answer Evidence has been put forward that the central glands are stimulated by oestrogens and the peripheral glands by androgens, thus an alteration in the ratio between androgens and oestrogens might account for benign prostatic hyperplasia.

Question What gross anatomical parts of the gland enlarge.

Answer The lateral lobes and the middle lobe.

Question Where is the middle lobe situated.

Answer In the midline above and between the plane through which the vasa deferens pass on their way to the crista urethralis.

Question Other than rectal examination and clinical experience what recent relatively simple measure has been described for the more accurate assessment of the size of the prostate.

Answer Transrectal ultrasonic examination. The normal prostate tends to have a triangular shape and is a symmetrical structure with a clearly defined capsule. Numerous fine homogeneous echoes are present, possibly caused by the periurethral glands. As the gland enlarges so the capsule assumes a more spherical configuration and the anterior/posterior diameter increases.

Question What changes may be seen on intravenous pyelography in prostatic obstruction.

Answer The bladder may be enlarged and trabeculated showing evidence of diverticular formation. It may be thick-walled and variable quantities of residual urine may be seen after voiding. Changes in the upper renal tract are rare unless the patient is suffering from chronic retention with overflow incontinence.

Question What might you suspect if a hydronephrosis is present without evidence of retention.

Answer Carcinoma of the prostate.

Question What are the chief complications of transurethral prostatectomy.

Answer

1 Perforation of the capsule. This is of little importance unless it is fairly large in which case leakage of irrigation fluid may occur into the periprostatic tissues or even into the peritoneal cavity. Either of these events may produce 'shock'. The pelvis should be explored and a drain left in the Cave of Retzius. If an intraperitoneal perforation has been caused the intestine must be carefully examined.

2 Electrolyte complications may follow the infusion of large volumes of glycine. This may produce bizarre neurological effects including epilepsy. The condition can be relieved by the administration of frusemide.

3 Secondary haemorrhage. This normally occurs on or about the 10th day and in a very small percentage of patients may be sufficient to produce clot retention.

4 Stricture formation. Common sites for the development of strictures following TUR are:

(a) within the meatus, usually 0.5 cm from the tip.

(b) peno-scrotal angle produced by angulation of the penis by the rigid instrument causing pressure necrosis.

(c) just below the external sphincter.

Many strictures can be avoided by performing a urethrotomy prior to commencing the operation if the urethra does not accept a 24 Ch sheath.

5 Incontinence. This complication may follow prostatectomy performed in the presence of some undiagnosed condition such as disseminated sclerosis but most follow resections which have inadvertently cut deeply into the tissues distal to the veru montanum.

6 Retrograde ejaculation.

7 Rarely epididymitis.

Comment Deep venous thrombosis followed by pulmonary embolism rarely follows transurethral prostatic resection in contrast to its relative frequency following retropubic or transvesical prostatectomy.

Physical examination on his present admission. This revealed no abnormality other than mild hypertension although his physical appearance suggested that a rapid weight loss had recently occurred. A vague swelling was palpable in the epigastrium.

Question What is the most reasonable diagnosis.

Answer In view of the loss of appetite, loss of weight and occasional vomiting a presumptive diagnosis of carcinoma of the stomach can be made.

Question What are the major symptoms associated with carcinoma of the stomach.

Answer Much depends upon the anatomical situation and the size and type of growth. Situated at the cardiac end of the stomach dysphagia eventually develops, situated on the antrum the symptoms of pyloric stenosis associated with vomiting and loss of weight. Tumours in the body of the stomach may cause an ill-defined dyspepsia which is eventually accompanied by anorexia.

Rarely the first evidence of a gastric cancer may be the presence of metastases, one of the classical sites being enlargement of the left supraclavicular lymph node.

A second factor is the macroscopic type of tumour. Thus patients suffering from gross infiltrative lesions producing the condition known as 'linitis plastica' frequently regurgitate their food rather than vomit. Ulcerative lesions of the body of the stomach may cause intractable ulcer type symptoms.

Question What investigations would be required to confirm the diagnosis.

Answer

1 Double contrast radiology. The result in this patient is shown in Figs 7.1 and 7.2

2 Endoscopy and biopsy of any gastric lesion found.

Question What additional investigations may prove useful.

Answer

1 Laparoscopy.

2 Ultrasonic investigation of the liver.

3 CAT.

4 Investigations necessary to determine the patient's fitness for surgery.

Question What do Figs 7.1 and 7.2 show.

Answer A large tumour occupying the pyloric end of the stomach.

Comment Endoscopy revealed a large antral tumour, biopsies of which showed a mucoid type of tumour. Laparoscopy showed that penetration of the serosal surface of the stomach had already occurred

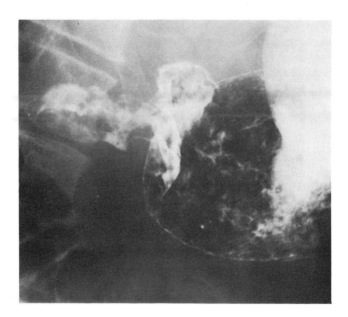

7.1

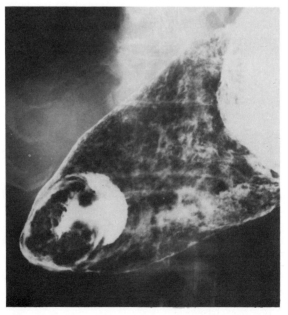

7.2

and obviously enlarged lymph nodes were present in the pyloric region. Ultrasonography of the liver showed no evidence of metastases. The chest X-ray showed no abnormality. The ECG showed an inverted T wave in Lead 1, in keeping with his previous cardiac history.

Question What operation, if any, is therefore possible.

Answer If anything at all is possible the only option will be some form of gastrectomy or gastroenterostomy.

Question What types of gastrectomy are commonly performed for this condition.

Answer Total gastrectomy or partial gastrectomy. Two forms of the latter have been described.

    (a) Bilroth gastrectomy.

    (b) Polya gastrectomy.

Both these operations were devised at the latter part of the nineteenth century.

Question Are there any contraindications other than the general condition of the patient which might dissuade a surgeon from performing a laparotomy followed by a palliative operation.

Answer Possibly the presence of widespread metastases in the absence of symptoms which can be alleviated by surgery.

Question What is the operability rate of carcinoma of the stomach using this term to include both palliative or potentially curative surgery.

Answer This varies in different series. In most series approximately 80 per cent of patients are deemed to be operable. However, of the patients operated upon only approximately 50 per cent have resectable tumours.

Question If the tumour is found to be unresectable what surgical alternative exists.

Answer A lesser procedure such as a gastroenterostomy might be possible. However, this may have to be 'fashioned'. The ideal site for a gastroenterostomy is on a line to the right of a vertical plane from the hiatus. However, in the presence of a large antral tumour it may be impossible to achieve such a position for the stoma and an anterior gastroenterostomy may have to be constructed with the anastomosis placed high on the anterior surface of the stomach.

Question What is the difference between the Bilroth and the Polya type of operation.

Answer In the Bilroth procedure intestinal continuity is restored by a direct anastomosis between the gastric remnant and the duodenum whereas in the Polya type gastrectomy the duodenum is closed and intestinal continuity restored by anastomosing the gastric remnant to the proximal jejunum.

Question Which operation is preferable in patients suffering from cancer of the stomach.

Answer Probably the Polya type since the Bilroth anastomosis can become rapidly blocked by local extension of the disease from pyloric lymph nodes if these have been left *in situ*.

Question What is meant by the term radical R_2/R_3 gastrectomy.

Answer This term is applied to the procedure described for dealing with gastric cancer by the Japanese Research Society for Gastric Cancer. For antral lesions a distal two-thirds subtotal gastrectomy is performed together with clearance of the perigastric nodes and the nodes along the left gastric and coeliac axis arteries and nodes in the hepato-duodenal ligament. For lesions elsewhere in the stomach a total gastrectomy is performed removing the lower 5 cm of the oesophagus, accompanied by clearance of the above mentioned node groups together with a subtotal pancreatectomy and splenectomy followed by removal of any nodes found along the common hepatic and splenic arteries.

Such radical surgery is only performed when the tumour is confined to the wall of stomach with minimal serosal involvement. In addition there must be no evidence of hepatic metastases, no peritoneal metastases and nodal involvement, if present, must not extent to the hepato-duodenal, retropancreatic or para-aortic areas.

Question What major early complications are associated with these operations.

Answer The Bilroth I type of gastrectomy may leak from the site on the lesser curve at which it is anastomosed to the upper border of the duodenum. The chief immediate danger associated with a Polya gastrectomy is rupture of the duodenal stump, although this is considerably more common following the closure of a duodenum in which severe duodenal ulceration is present

Question What is the anticipated mortality following gastric resection in patients suffering from carcinoma of the stomach.

Answer The mortality rises rapidly with advancing age. Over 70 years of age mortality rates as high as 30 per cent have been reported. Proximal gastrectomy has a higher mortality than distal gastrectomy and the operative mortality of total gastrectomy is higher than either of these lesser operations.

Question What are the chief factors influencing the prognosis.

Answer

1 Tumour size.

2 Depth of invasion. Serosal involvement is associated with a negligible five year survival.

3 Lymph node metastases which are themselves more common once serosal invasion has occurred.

4 Tumour site. Patients suffering from cardiac tumours have a significantly worse prognosis than patients suffering from cancers of the body and antrum.

Question Has chemotherapy any part to play in the treatment of carcinoma of the stomach when metastatic disease is associated with this tumour.

Answer Little benefit appears to follow the use of chemotherapeutic agents but some objective response has been reported using 5-Fluorouracil, *bis* chlorethyl nitrosourea (BCNU), Adriamycin and Mitomycin C although the ultimate prognosis does not appear to be improved.

Question Is there a geographical variation in the incidence of cancer of the stomach.

Answer Yes. There is a thirtyfold difference between the incidence of gastric cancer in Japan as compared to the incidence in the white population of the United States.

Question Does this apply to all types of cancer of the stomach.

Answer According to some histopathologists this extraordinary variability is ascribed only to the intestinal type of cancer of the stomach whilst no variation in incidence is found in the diffuse type.

Question Who first classified cancer of the stomach into these two major histopathological types.

Answer The Finnish pathologists, Lauren and Jarvi in 1951.

Question What are the chief histological features which distinguish these two types of tumour.

Answer The intestinal type of cancer of the stomach has a glandular pattern accompanied by papillary formation or solid components. Any secretion present tends to be chiefly in the glandular lumina. The diffuse type is made up of scattered solitary or small clusters of cells, glandular lumina being uncommon or, if present, small and indefinite. According to Lauren, of the 1344 tumours examined one-half were of the intestinal type, one-third diffuse and the remainder unclassifiable.

Question What other histological classification has been proposed.

Answer That by Mulligan and Rember in 1974. They described three main types of cancer of the stomach: the mucous cell cancer comprising about a half of the tumours they examined, which is equivalent to the intestinal cancer type of cancer described by Lauren and Jorvi; the pylorocardiac gland cell carcinoma comprising one-quarter; and the intestinal cell cancer, also comprising one-quarter of all cases.

Question What is the chief difference between these two classifications.

Answer The recognition by Mulligan and Rember of pylorocardiac gland carcinomata which are chiefly situated, as one would expect, in the antrum or cardia. However, many tumours are heterogeneous in structure.

Question Does the incidence of cancer of the stomach increase with age.

Answer Yes.

Question What is the sex incidence.

Answer Twice as many men are affected as women at every age.

Question Has the overall mortality from carcinoma of the stomach declined.

Answer Yes. This suggests a diminished exposure to whatever carcinogen is responsible for the disease. This decrease in mortality is not confined to a single country, the greatest reduction has been seen in the United States in which the mortality has decreased by half between 1950 and 1960. The least reduction in incidence has occurred in Japan where the decrease in mortality is only between 10 and 20 per cent.

Question What specific factors are known to be associated with gastric cancer.

Answer

1 Blood group. Whereas blood group O is associated with an increased incidence of duodenal ulceration blood group A is associated with a 20 per cent excess of gastric cancer in all areas.

2 Pernicious anaemia; gastric cancer is three times more common in patients suffering from pernicious anaemia than in normal individuals.

3 Type B chronic gastritis.

Question What is type B chronic gastritis.

Answer An atrophic gastritis in which the test for parietal cell antibody is negative, serum gastrin levels are low and the gastritis chiefly affects the antral mucosa.

4 A higher incidence of gastric cancer occurs in asbestos workers.

5 Diet. A survey performed in Hawaii in which there is an intermix between Japanese migrants, Hawaiian born Japanese and white Hawaiians of American origin suggests that the risk of the disease is increased about twofold by a diet consisting of dried and salted fish and pickled vegetables as compared to a Western type of diet.

6 Previous benign gastric ulceration. Once considered common, the importance of benign gastric ulceration as a precursor of malignancy is now considered rare.

Question What chemical carcinogen is a possible cause of carcinoma of the stomach.

Answer Nitroso-compounds which occur naturally in many foods especially meat and fish. The hypothesis that N-nitroso compounds might be a cause of cancer is based on their known carcinogenicity and the fact that they may be formed *in vivo* in the stomach by a reaction between nitrites and secondary amines and N-substituted amines. Nitrites are added as preservatives to foods such as bacon and are formed from nitrates in the saliva by bacterial action.

Question What is meant by the term 'early gastric cancer'.

Answer The term 'early gastric cancer', EGC, was coined by the Japanese, in whom gastric cancer is the commonest form of malignant disease, to describe gastric cancers limited to the mucosa and submucosa regardless of whether lymph node involvement is present or not.

Question What are the basic patterns of EGC.

Answer Three basic patterns are recognized:

Type I Protruded type

Type II
- 11a superficial type
- elevated type   } Elevated lesion   13%
- 11b Flat type   76%

Type III
- 11c Depressed type   } Depressed lesion   11%
- Excavated type

This classification is that proposed by the Japanese Research Society for Gastric Cancer.

Question What types of growth pattern are recognized.

Answer

1 The superficial spreading lesion is a tumour having a diameter of over 4 cm and is either confined to the mucosa or only partly invading the submucosa.

2 The penetrating type which has a diameter of less than 4 cm but which is invading the submucosa in a wide penetrating fashion. This type of tumour can be further divided into:

(a) Type A, in which the tumour is invading expansively through the muscularis mucosa.

(b) Type B, in which the tumour is growing in an infiltrative manner.

A third type is also described known as the small mucosal type which is less than 4 cm in diameter and can be classified as neither superficial or penetrating.

Question What histological pattern is associated with early gastric cancer.

Answer The histological pattern of EGC appears to depend upon the age of the patient. In young adults, i.e. 30 years of age or less the lesion is usually poorly differentiated whereas in the older patient such tumours are moderately to well differentiated. A further difference appears to be an absence of mucosal change peripheral to the tumour in the younger patient whereas in the older patient moderate to severe intestinal metaplasia is commonly present.

Question What is the clinical importance of EGC.

Answer EGC is potentially curable; 5 year survival rates in excess of 80 per cent have been reported by the Japanese whereas the combination of a penetrating lesion together with lymph node involvement is associated with five year survival rate of 15 per cent or less.

Question What is the duration of survival of patients suffering from gastric cancer following a palliative procedure.

Answer Rarely over six months.

Comment This patient was treated by a palliative Polya gastrectomy and within four months was readmitted suffering from malignant cachexia. The report on the specimen read as follows: A poorly differentiated adenocarcinoma arising from and ulcerating the gastric mucosa and invading through the gastric wall into the serosa. There is sufficient mucin production to warrant the descriptive term 'mucoid carcinoma'. There is widespread serosal involvement. Two of the three greater curve lymph nodes are involved by tumour and in addition there are several separate tumour deposits in the fat along the greater and lesser curvatures of the stomach.

Question What is the cause of malignant cachexia.

Answer This is not yet fully elucidated. It may be associated with simple anorexia leading to deficient food intake or it may be caused by simple obstruction making it impossible for the patient to eat. However, malignant cachexia is frequently associated with a low metabolic rate, the converse of the situation found in starvation. There is also some evidence that there is interference with the normal metabolism of the host, possibly caused by tumour derived products known as 'toxo-hormones'.

8

A male patient aged 49 was admitted complaining of upper abdominal 'dyspepsia' of 20 years duration. He described the pain in the following terms, in the early period the pain had been in the centre of the epigastrium and burning in character. It had always been episodic occurring at irregular intervals throughout the entire period. Once present, the pain had tended to be cyclical, developing when hungry or waking him at night. Each attack had lasted for several weeks and as time had progressed the pain had lost its periodicity and become widespread, being present in the back as well as in the epigastrium. As the attacks had become more severe he had begun to vomit, vomiting tending to temporarily relieve the pain.

Previous medical history This was negative other than the history given above.

Physical examination All systems were normal but examination of the abdomen revealed:

1 tenderness on palpation to the right of the epigastrium.

2 a succession splash.

Social habits The patient was a moderate drinker and smoked approximately 20 cigarettes a day.

Question What would be your presumptive diagnosis.

Answer Active duodenal ulceration complicated by pyloric stenosis or intermittent spasm.

Question What is the incidence of duodenal ulceration in Great Britain.

Answer Between the years 1930 and 1949 by studying autopsy figures, Watkinson found that the incidence of active duodenal ulceration was 5.5 per cent in males and 1.5 per cent in females. However, these figures probably now need considerable modification because the incidence of duodenal ulceration appears to have been slowly declining since these figures were first published. Furthermore, whilst in the past the major socio-economic group affected was Group 1 it is now more common in Group V.

Question What is the cause of duodenal ulceration.

Answer There are two significant causal factors:

1 the amount of acid and pepsin secreted.

2 breakdown of the physical and chemical protection of the mucosa.

Question Why can it be said with absolute certainty that acid plays a major role in the development of duodenal ulceration.

Answer Because duodenal ulceration never occurs in achlorhydric patients. However, 50 per cent of patients suffering from duodenal ulceration have acid levels in the normal range although they are at the upper end of this range. In contrast gastric ulceration occurs in patients who have acid levels within normal limits. Thus in considering peptic ulceration as opposed to duodenal ulceration two other factors, i.e. pepsin and mucosal resistance must also be considered.

Question What subsidiary factors have been identified.

Answer

1 Genetic factors:

(a) duodenal ulceration is more common in patients of blood group O who are non-secretors of ABO antigens.

(b) siblings of duodenal ulcer patients are some three times more likely to develop duodenal ulceration than unrelated controls.

2 Age, duodenal ulceration becomes relatively more common with advancing age. Twenty per cent of endoscopically proven ulcers occur beyond the age of 60.

3 Diet. The low masticatory diet of Southern India is associated with a higher incidence of peptic ulceration than the harder, wheat based diet of Northern India. One explanation advanced for this finding is that with high masticatory diets more saliva is swallowed. This inhibits gastric emptying and hence exposure of the duodenum to gastric acid.

4 Associated disease: there is an association between duodenal ulceration and:

(a) chronic renal failure.

(b) hyperparathyroidism.

(c) cirrhosis.

(d) chronic respiratory disease.

Question In order to confirm your clinical impression what investigations would you require.

Answer

1 Double contrast barium radiology. This investigation has a combined 20 per cent incidence of false positive and false negative results. It still remains difficult for the radiologist to demonstrate an ulcer crater particularly when there is gross scarring and deformity from long standing disease.

2 Endoscopy using small incremental doses of diazepam. This investigation is certainly superior to contrast radiology especially in patients suffering from an upper gastro-intestinal haemorrhage because it enables the clinician to identify the source of bleeding.

Question What are the classical radiological signs of duodenal ulceration.

Answer The normal duodenum adopts a shape commonly likened to a tricorn hat or the ace of spaces and the mucosal folds run parallel to its long axis. When a duodenal ulcer is active the pylorus may be seen by the radiologist to be in spasm. As the length of the history increases a trifolate or clover leaf deformity develops together with pseudodiverticulum formation. The great problem for the radiologist is to be able to demonstrate the ulcer crater itself either *en face* or *in profile*. The accuracy of a barium meal depends to a great extent on the radiologists experience as well as the changes which have taken place.

Question Would you perform gastric secretory tests.

Answer No, not as a routine. There are, however, two exceptions to this dogmatic negative.

Acid secretory studies are of assistance in the diagnosis of the Zollinger-Ellison syndrome and can also help to establish the cause of recurrent ulceration.

Question Which gastric secretory tests are in common use.

Answer

1 Tests involving stimulation of the parietal cell. This is normally achieved by stimulation with:
   (a) Pentagastrin, an analogue of gastrin.
   (b) Insulin.
   (c) A variety of meals.

2 Measurement of gastrin secretion.

Question What do gastric secretory tests measure.

Answer

1 The Basal Acid Output of the unstimulated stomach.

2 The Maximal Acid Output after stimulation. This is normally measured by collecting four consecutive 15 minute samples of gastric secretion, after the administration of 6 μg/kg of pentagastrin by intramuscular injection.

Question What are the values of basal secretion.

Answer In a normal subject approximately 2 mmol of HCl/h is secreted, this value increasing with weight and decreasing with advancing age. In patients suffering from a duodenal ulcer this value approaches 5 mmol/h or higher and in the Zollinger-Ellison syndrome 15 mmol/h.

Question What are the anticipated values for maximal acid secretion.

Answer In a normal individual maximal acid secretion rarely exceeds 20–30 mmol/h or 0.4 mmol/kg whereas in approximately 40 per cent of patients suffering from duodenal ulceration values in excess of 40 mmol/h are found, i.e. greater than 0.5 mmol/kg.

Question What is the Zollinger-Ellison syndrome.

Answer The Zollinger-Ellison syndrome is caused by either:

1 the presence of a gastrin secreting islet cell tumour of the pancreas.

2 G-cell hyperplasia of the antral area of the stomach. Gastrin secreting tumours of the pancreas are frequently associated with other endocrine tumours. Thus hyperplasia or true adenomata of the parathyroid and anterior hypophysis may occur synchronously or sequentially. This constellation is known as the MEN I syndrome. If this occurs as an autosomal dominant disorder, tumours of the islet cells other than those producing gastrin may occur in the pancreas producing the Werner-Morrison syndrome in which the major clinical feature is diarrhoea of such severity that hypokalaemia occurs.

Question What are the major clinical features of the Zollinger-Ellison syndrome.

Answer

1 Severe intractable ulceration in the first part of the duodenum and beyond.

2 Rapid development of recurrent ulceration after apparently adequate surgery.

3 Severe diarrhoea caused by the failure of the excessive amounts of acid secreted to be neutralized by the alkaline duodenal and pancreatic juices. In addition, true steatorrhoea may occur due to acid inactivation of the pancreatic lipase and the precipitation of bile salts.

4 Bilateral oedema of the legs due to a protein losing enteropathy.

Question What constellation of endocrine tumours form the MEN II syndrome.

Answer The MEN II syndrome consists of the triad parathyroid adenoma, medullary carcinoma of the thyroid and phaeochromocytoma.

There is also a variant of this syndrome known as the MEN II B or MEN III in which hyperparathyroidism is rare. The chief features of this last syndrome are the presence of a medullary carcinoma of the thyroid and a phaeochromocytoma together with multiple mucosal neuromata with or without a Marfanoid habitus.

Comment In the only patient suffering from the Zollinger-Ellison syndrome that the author has seen he performed a partial gastrectomy, in ignorance of the true diagnosis, the syndrome not having been described, and within 14 days the patient had already developed severe anastomotic ulceration.

Question What is the chief use of the insulin test.

Answer The chief use of the insulin test is to test the adequacy of vagotomy.

Question What is the eponymous name given to the insulin test.

Answer The Hollander Test.

Question How is this test conducted.

Answer Basal gastric secretion is collected for four consecutive 15 minute periods. 0.2 units of insulin/kg of body weight is then administered intravenously and aspiration continued for a further eight consecutive 15 minute periods. Each sample is tested by titration up to pH 7.0. The test is positive when the acidity increases more than 20 mmol/l above the basal level in any 15 minute period unless the basal level is zero in which case an increase of 10 mmol/l is sufficient to be deemed positive. A blood glucose level below 2.8 mmol/l (45 mg/100 ml) is necessary to ensure a positive response.

'Early' and 'Late' positive responses have also been recognized, the former being somewhat more significant than the latter. An early positive response during which more than 20 mmol/h of acid are secreted implies residual innervation and, therefore, an incomplete vagotomy.

Question How is the plasma gastrin level measured.

Answer By radio immunoassay.

Question What are the chief stimulators of gastrin secretion.

Answer The presence of protein in the antrum or distension of antrum. When the pH within the antrum falls gastrin release is inhibited due to negative feedback control.

Question What types of stimulator are used to estimate changes in the plasma gastrin concentration.

Answer Protein meals, calcium infusion and secretin.

Question In what condition does the plasma gastrin rise dramatically.

Answer In the presence of a gastrin secreting islet cell tumour of the pancreas.

Question What is meant by the term mucosal barrier.

Answer The mucosal barrier is a physiological concept involving the mechanisms by which the mucosa keeps hydrogen ions within the lumen of the gut and prevents their back diffusion to the epithelial lining and at the same time prevents sodium ions diffusing into the lumen from the mucosa.

Question What is the composition of the mucus layer.

Answer The mucus layer consists of two phases. The inner layer lying on the surface of the mucosa is a gel, the principle functions of which are to protect the epithelium from the noxious action of acid/pepsin and bile. It is composed of cross-linking glycoprotein subunits. The water within this gel confines the HCO_3 within it so that H^+ ion back diffusing into the mucus is progressively neutralized. Lying on the superficial surface of the gel is a liquid phase which is primarily a lubricant containing glycoprotein subunits from the broken down gel mucus.

The formation of the protective gel depends upon the renewal of the mucus secreting cells of the surface epithelium, these cells being derived from cells deep in the crypts. Factors decreasing the renewal of mucosal cells by increasing epithelial cell loss include the non-steroidal anti-inflammatory agents. Factors which diminish the efficacy of the mucosal barrier include aspirin, alcohol and the bile salts, all of which increase ionic permeability.

Question Is the presence of duodenal ulceration necessarily associated with symptoms.

Answer No. Endoscopic follow-up studies have shown that some 50 per cent of early ulcer relapses are asymptomatic.

Question Does this pose difficulties.

Answer Yes, because the loss of symptoms following any form of treatment is not necessarily a guarantee of cure.

Comment During the 20 years this patient had suffered he had received a variety of medical treatments. In the early period this had chiefly consisted of periods of bedrest during which various diets, antacids and anticholinergic drugs had been prescribed. Latterly, however, he had been treated first with cimetidine and then with ranitidine.

Question What are cimetidine and ranitidine.

Answer These drugs attach themselves to the H_2 receptors on the parietal cell and inhibit both basal and nocturnal acid secretion and also the acid response to:

1 food.
2 vagal stimulation.
3 gastrin or pentagastrin stimulation.
4 histamine and its analogues.

Question In which organs are H_2 receptors found.

Answer Stomach, uterus and heart

Question In what organs are H_1 receptors found.

Answer Skin, bronchi and nasal mucus membranes.

Question Who confirmed the presence of H_2 receptors.

Answer Black and his co-workers at Smith, Kline and French in 1972. The first H_2 receptor antagonist to be synthesized was buramide, later replaced by metiamide which was abandoned because of severe side effects to be replaced by cimetidine. In turn, this last mentioned drug manufactured by Smith, Kline and French has been largely replaced by ranitidine (Zantac, Glaxo).

Question What, if any, are the advantages of ranitidine over cimetidine.

Answer Ranitidine is eight times more potent than cimetidine in inhibiting histamine induced acid secretion and four to five times more effective in inhibiting physiological secretion. It also lacks the anti-androgenic effects of cimetidine.

Question What is the normal prescribed dose of ranitidine.

Answer 150 mg bd. A twice daily dose is recommended since after one dose gastric secretion is suppressed for approximately 12 hours.

Question What other drug has also been used with somewhat better results than simple antacid or placebo therapy.

Answer Sucralfate, dose 1 g four times a day. Some trials have shown that this drug is equally as effective as the H_2 antagonists in the treatment of duodenal and gastric ulceration.

Question What is the quantitative reduction in acid secretion achieved by the H_2 blockers.

Answer In Europeans the reduction in acid secretion varies from 50 to 70 per cent which is approximately equal to the effect produced by vagotomy.

Question What do double blind trials reveal as to the effectiveness of H_2 antagonists.

Answer They reveal that whereas with a placebo the satisfactory response varies between 20 and 70 per cent according to the country in which the trial takes place, treatment with H_2 antagonists produces an almost universal response rate of between 60 and 70 per cent.

Question What is the action of sucralfate.

Answer The action of this drug is not fully understood. It is believed that it may inhibit the action of pepsin partly by direct absorption and partly by forming complexes with proteins that would otherwise be digested by pepsin. A second action is believed to be the lessening of back diffusion of H ion.

Question What is the relapse rate of duodenal ulcers following cessation of medical therapy.

Answer Approximately 70 per cent. If therapy is continued for a period of one year recent trials have shown that ranitidine is superior to cimetidine. At the end of 12 months after the termination of maintenance therapy, 23 per cent of patients maintained on ranitidine have relapsed as compared to 37 per cent of patients maintained for one year on cimetidine. These results were obtained by performing an endoscopy at four monthly intervals following the cessation of treatment.

Even if either drug is continued after healing has been achieved a recent American study has shown that a relapse rate of some 16 per cent can be expected during a period of one year's maintenance therapy.

Comment Study of various papers dealing with the immediate treatment and the maintenance of therapy once healing has been achieved suggest that the H_2 antagonists do not substantially or favourably alter the natural history of peptic ulceration which is a relapsing disease. However, many observers have concluded that duodenal ulceration is a self-limiting disease which, if survived, without complications for a period of several years, tends to pass into spontaneous remission. Certainly this was the author's personal experience until his natural history was interrupted by open heart surgery.

Question What are the chief indications for surgical treatment in duodenal ulceration.

Answer

1 *Intractability*

This term can now be interpreted as frequent relapse following adequate maintenance therapy associated with an inability of the patient to cope with the situation or the symptoms.

2 *Bleeding*

The probability of massive haemorrhage from a duodenal ulcer varies considerably according to the series examined. According to estimates made at the Cleveland University Hospital, USA, once bleeding has occurred a further haemorrhage can be expected in 23 per cent within three years and in 50 per cent by the tenth year. The estimate of the chances of a first bleed are between 20 and 25 per cent.

Question What factors govern the mortality associated with bleeding.

Answer The three major factors influencing mortality are:

1 The age of the patient and associated cardiovascular disease.

2 The severity of the bleed.

3 Repeated bleeding.

Question How would you treat massive repeated bleeding in a male over 50 years of age.

Answer Assuming there was no contra-indication, by surgery. The alternative surgical approaches include:

1 Partial gastrectomy.

2 Pyloroplasty followed by oversewing of the ulcer and 'vagotomy'. The operative mortality of partial gastrectomy is higher in all series than the immediate mortality of vagotomy and pyloroplasty. However, rebleeding following partial gastrectomy is somewhat less than that following vagotomy, pyloroplasty and oversewing of the ulcer.

3 Recently reports have appeared in the literature suggesting that

a satisfactory result can be achieved in elderly patients by the use of VAG laser therapy. This treatment is delivered by means of a fibreoptic endoscope. A significant number of ulcers cannot, however, be treated in this manner because the ulcer cannot be visualized 'en face'. The laser beam is not directed at the open vessel itself but at the surrounding tissue so that shrinkage will result in blockage of the offending artery.

Question What is the estimated mortality of a bleed from a chronic peptic ulcer.

Answer Ten per cent at the first bleed, 20 per cent at the second and between 30 and 40 per cent if persistent uncontrolled haemorrhage occurs.

3 *Perforation*

The treatment of perforation remains a matter for debate. The classical manner of treatment is to open the abdomen and perform a simple suture. However, many surgeons have drawn attention to the fact that when the abdomen is opened the perforation is nearly always sealed. Furthermore, it has been pointed out that simple suture of subacute ulcers with a history of less than three months is followed, in a proportion of cases, by intractable symptoms. It has, therefore, been argued that perforation following a short history can be treated as well, if not better, conservatively, i.e. by the administration of analgesics and simple naso-gastric suction together with ranitidine intravenously and that if perforation occurs following a long history of ulcer dyspepsia it should be treated by a definitive operation.

Question What is the mortality associated with perforation.

Answer Between 5 and 15 per cent depending on the series examined.

Question What lethal complication directly associated with the ulcer itself may follow simple suture.

Answer Reperforation may occur, although this is rare; bleeding is more common.

Question Is the mortality of definite surgery in the presence of a perforation greater than that associated with simple suture.

Answer No, in many series it is somewhat lower. However, the better results in terms of operative mortality achieved by definitive surgery may be obtained because good risk patients tend to be treated by more complex operations and the bad risk patients by simpler procedures.

4 *Stenosis*

Obstruction due to duodenal ulceration is usually the result of previous scarring together with oedema, the latter possibly being precipitated by recurrent ulceration. It may be associated with gross electrolyte imbalance caused by the severe vomiting which may lead to dehydration and alkalosis both of which require correction prior to surgery. The presence of obstructive symptoms is an absolute indication for surgical intervention.

Comment This patient suffering from obstructive symptoms and a long history of ulcer dyspepsia was treated by truncal vagotomy and posterior gastroenterostomy.

Question What is the effect of vagotomy on acid secretion.
Answer
 1 Basal acid output is reduced by some 80–90 per cent.
 2 Maximal acid secretion, induced by pentagastrin stimulation; by 50 to 60 per cent.
Similar results follow truncal vagotomy with drainage (TVD), selective vagotomy, and posterior truncal vagotomy accompanied by anterior seromyotomy.

Question What alternative procedures have been described.
Answer
 1 Simple posterior gastroenterostomy. This operation was abandoned when it was shown that in about 50 per cent of patients anastomotic ulceration developed in the efferent loop.
 2 Highly selective vagotomy associated with dilatation of the stenotic segment.

Question What are the advantages of highly selective vagotomy (HSV) over truncal vagotomy (TV).
Answer Two major advantages have been claimed for HSV as compared to TV. They are:
 1 that truncal vagotomy is followed by diarrhoea in a variable number of patients, figures varying between 2 and 68 per cent having been quoted in the literature. However, much depends on the observers interpretation of the term diarrhoea. Severe episodic diarrhoea which may be accompanied by incontinence probably affects no more than three per cent of all patients subjected to truncal vagotomy regardless of the method of drainage, and persistent diarrhoea, defined as the passage of six or more unformed stools daily, is even rarer.
 2 that truncal vagotomy followed by a drainage procedure is followed in a larger percentage of patients by 'dumping'. Figures for the difference in the incidence of this syndrome varies according to the series examined between four and eight per cent for HSV and 20 and 30 per cent for TVD.

Comment Despite these apparent advantages when the overall results were examined by Clark *et al.* (1968) *British Journal of Surgery.* **73.** they found that the Visick grading of their two groups of patients, one group treated by TVD and the other by HSV without drainage was not significantly different. TVD was followed by 78.5 per cent patients in Visick's group I and II and HSV by 78.3 per cent patients in this category.

Question Are there any possible disadvantages to HSV.

Answer It is not yet clear what the eventual ulcer recurrence rate will be following HSV. It appears from the literature that the early reports erred on an optimistic side. Recently, recurrence rates as high as 14 per cent have been quoted in the literature. However, the majority of these can be adequately controlled by the use of ranitidine and, therefore, do not necessarily require further operation.

Question How would you classify the complications of gastric surgery.

Answer

1 Complications associated with enterogastric reflux:

(a) Bile vomiting.

(b) Biliary gastritis.

(c) Oesophagitis due to gastro-oesophageal reflux.

2 Complications associated with rapid emptying of the stomach or gastric remnant:

(a) Diarrhoea.

(b) Dumping.

(c) Malabsorption, leading to steatorrhoea, anaemia and bone disease.

(d) Post-prandial hypoglycaemia.

3 Complications associated with gastric retention.

(a) Vomiting.

(b) Gastric ulceration.

(c) Bezoar formation.

4 Complications associated with changes in biliary tract physiology, especially associated with truncal vagotomy, e.g. gall-stones.

Comment This patient, seen one year following surgery was classified as a Visick I.

9

A female, aged 72, presented complaining of intermittent attacks of diarrhoea over the past 13 months. On occasions her bowels had been opened as much as seven times a day. No mucus or blood had been noted by the patient at any time. Approximately two weeks prior to her clinic appointment she had suffered an ill localized attack of upper abdominal pain radiating to the back which had been relieved by pethidine. Over a period of one month she had complained of generalized itching and three weeks prior to her appointment she had suffered from intermittent nausea and had vomited on two occasions. She had never observed any change in the colour of her conjunctivae.

Previous medical history. Aged 47, hysterectomy for fibroids. Aged 50, fracture of the right hip, treated by open reduction. Aged 53, found to have hypertension, present medication oxyprenolol hydrochloride (Trasidrex, Ciba) tabs one daily and potassium chloride (Slow K, Ciba). A recent complaint of 'rheumatism' had led to treatment by the non-steroidal anti-inflammatory drugs, indomethacin (Indocid, Morson) and ibuprofen (Brufen, Boots).

Question Can the medication prescribed above result in any surgical complications.

Answer

1 Potassium chloride may cause ulceration and strictures of the small bowel. It should not be given in patients known to have gastro-intestinal conditions such as Crohn's disease. If held up in the small bowel perforation may follow mucosal ulceration.

2 Both the non-steroidal anti-inflammatory drugs prescribed may produce gastrointestinal disturbance and pruritis. In addition, both may result in gastric ulceration, this more commonly occurring after medication with indomethacin than ibuprofen. Both may produce non-specific gastrointestinal disturbance.

Physical Examination

Inspection revealed

1 a yellowish tinge of the conjunctivae.
2 a surgical scar on the abdomen.
3 a surgical scar over the right thigh, measurement of the legs showed that the right leg was 1½" shorter than the left.

Abdominal examination	palpation revealed no masses.
	P.R. negative.
Respiratory system	No abnormality.
Central nervous system	No abnormality.
Cardiovascular system	B.P. 140/90 No cardiac enlargement.

Question In view of the history and the trace of jaundice found on clinical examination what investigations would you initially order.

Answer

1 Ultrasound examination of the biliary tract.

2 Liver function tests, the most important of which are:
   (a) serum bilirubin.
   (b) alkaline phosphatase.
   (c) serum alanine transferase (SGPT)

Comment The following results were received:

1 Ultrasonography revealed a solitary stone in the gall bladder, the common bile duct measured 9 mm in diameter.

2 Serum bilirubin 81 μmol/l (normal value 5–17 μmol/l). Alkaline Phosphatase 553 U/l (normal value 24–104). Serum alanine transferase (SGPT) 242 U/l (normal value, up to 42).

Question Does the ultrasound result assist in making a specific diagnosis.

Answer No. Although the recent attack of upper abdominal pain may have been caused by the calculus demonstrated in the gall bladder it is unlikely that it could produce the severe disturbance of the serum enzymes. However, occasionally a large calculus can impact in the neck of the gall bladder and provoke such a severe degree of inflammatory oedema that the common duct is transiently obstructed. The ultrasound does demonstrate, however, that there must be some obstruction to the lower end of the common bile duct since the maximal diameter of a normal duct as measured by ultrasonography is 6 mm.

Question What is the origin of the bilirubin normally found in the plasma.

Answer Eighty per cent is the end product of haem and the remainder is derived from myoglobin and some of the respiratory enzymes. Unconjugated bilirubin is only lipid soluble. It is converted to a water soluble compound by conjugation and excreted into the bile as bilirubin diglucuronide.

Question Does the bilirubin level continue to rise in the presence of complete obstruction to the bile ducts.

Answer No. Normally the serum bilirubin rises rapidly but after about

77

three weeks even in the presence of continued obstruction it levels off, possibly due to excretion of bile pigment by the kidney and the passage of unconjugated bilirubin through the intestinal mucosa to the gut.

Question In this patient the alkaline phosphatase is grossly elevated 553 U/l; what is the significance of this.

Answer Alkaline phosphatase is a phosphomonoesterase. Elevation to this level suggests that the jaundice in this patient is cholestatic (post-hepatic) rather than hepatic in origin. Alkaline phosphatase has a half-life in the serum of seven days and as a result it tends to remain elevated after the serum bilirubin has returned to normal, a point well illustrated in this particular patient. However, this investigation is non-specific in the sense that the obstructing agent does not necessarily have to be situated in or around the extrahepatic ductal system. Thus a raised alkaline phosphatase may be found when amyloid disease affects the liver, in multiple liver abscesses and leukaemic deposits presumably due to obstruction of the intrahepatic bile channels.

Question What is the significance of the raised serum alanine transferase.

Answer The circulating level of this enzyme in the serum is raised in both cholestasis and hepato-cellular disease. It parallels the serum alkaline phosphatase in cholestasis and thus confirms that this enzyme is of hepato-biliary origin.

Question Can other conditions cause a raised serum alkaline phosphatase.

Answer Yes, chiefly bone diseases.

Comment Biochemical assessment suggests the presence of extrahepatic obstruction. The recent attack of pain requiring the administration of pethidine for its relief suggests an attack of biliary colic. However, the long history of intermittent diarrhoea requires explanation.

Question Could the diarrhoea of which the patient complains be explained on the basis of a pancreato-biliary pathology.

Answer Yes, but one would have to assume either that complete obstruction of the common bile duct was present leading to an absence of bile salts in the gastro-intestinal tract or that the pancreatic duct was blocked leading to an absence of lipase in the gut. In either event the result would be the onset of steatorrhoea. Since this patient did not describe the typical stools of steatorrhoea which are characteristically bulky and foul smelling either condition is unlikely.

Question Since the biochemical findings are undoubtedly those of cholestasis what other investigations may assist in reaching a definitive diagnosis.

Answer Oral cholangiography, using Idopace, is of no assistance in this patient since the concentration of dye is insufficient to produce satisfactory definition of the biliary tract when the serum bilirubin is above 34 μmol/l. Similarly intravenous cholangiography using Ioglycamide is unsatisfactory when the bilirubin concentration is above 68 μmol/l.

Therefore resort must be made to endoscopic-cholangiopancreatography (ERCP) if this investigation is technically possible.

Question How is this investigation performed.

Answer The patient is lightly sedated with atropine and diazepam and duodenal motility is reduced by the intermittent intravenous administration of hyoscine N-butylbromide (Buscopan, Boerhringer Ingelheim). An Olympus JFB2 fibrescope is passed into the duodenum and the papilla identified. Under direct vision a cannula is introduced and contrast medium introduced, first into the biliary tree and then into the pancreatic duct.

Question Are any precautions necessary prior to this manoeuvre.

Answer In view of the suspected biliary obstruction 80 mg of gentamicin and 250 mg of ampicillin should be administered four hours before the procedure.

Question What are the complications associated with ERCP.

Answer

1 If the dye is injected into an infected biliary tree without the prior administration of antibiotics a febrile reaction or septicaemia may occur.

2 Acute pancreatitis. A rise in the serum amylase is relatively common after this procedure but a clinical attack of pancreatitis is fortunately rare. Some investigators have suggested that acute pancreatitis is more common if small repeated doses of dye are injected into the pancreas rather than a single bolus.

Comment The result of this investigation are shown in Figs 9.1 and 9.2.

Question What do they show.

Answer Figure 9.1 shows:

(a) at least two large facetted stones in the lower end of the common bile duct (1)

(b) a smaller stone impacted in the ampullary region (3)

(c) a normal pancreatic duct (2)

Figure 9.2 shows:

(a) the valve of Heister within the cystic duct (4)

(b) a large solitary stone lying in the fundus of the gall bladder (5)

Question In view of the absence of contraindications what would you advise.

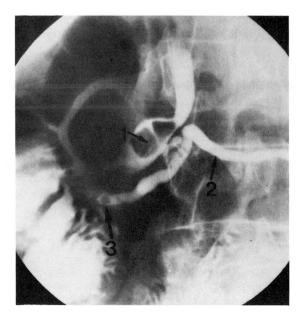

9.1

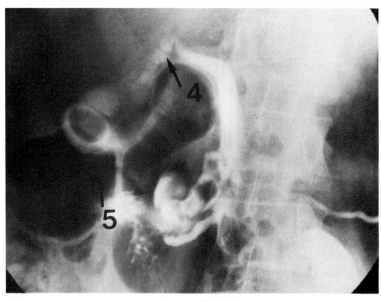

9.2

Answer Cholecystectomy and exploration of the common bile duct.

Question Is any further investigation necessary before surgery in this patient.

Answer Yes, it is essential to establish that the prothrombin time is within normal limits. In this patient the prothrombin time measured 13 sec, (normal value 12 sec).

Question In view of the diagnosis of obstructive jaundice would you consider the administration of prophylactic antibiotics.

Answer Yes, an antibiotic is required which is active against both coliforms and the staphylococci. A cephalosporin such as cephazolin would be adequate. An intramuscular injection of this drug produces a peak plasma concentration of 30 µg or more per ml within one hour. A recommended dose is 1 g intramuscularly one hour prior to surgery and 500 mg eight hourly for five days. The incidence of wound sepsis has been shown to be reduced from approximately 17 per cent to three per cent using this antibiotic regime.

Comment The abdomen was opened using a right paramedian incision. No calculi could be palpated in the common bile duct but having opened the duct along its vertical axis, in passing the Desjardin forceps in a caudal direction soft biliary debris was obtained. No stone was removed which corresponded in shape to the shadows seen on the radiographs. After repeatedly irrigating the duct a Bakes dilator was passed, apparently into the duodenum but on re-irrigating the duct fluid was seen to be escaping into the peripancreatic areolar tissues. A cholangiogram was then performed (Fig. 9.3).

Question What are the absolute clinical indications to explore the common bile duct.

Answer

1   The presence of jaundice at the time of operation.

2   A dilated biliary tree.

3   The presence of a palpable stone.

Secondary indications for exploration are:

1   The presence of multiple small stones in gall bladder.

2   A previous history of jaundice.

3   A history of pancreatitis.

Question What does Fig. 9.3 show.

Answer

1   No entry of dye into the duodenum.

2   The longer arrow may indicate either residual debris in the lower end of the common bile duct, or, the tract of the false passage produced by the passage of the Bakes dilator.

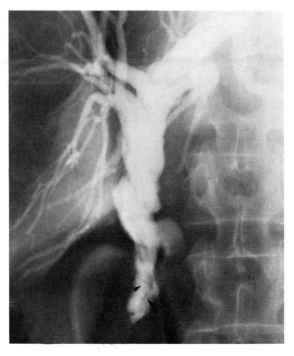

9.3

3 A long cystic duct, at this time the gall bladder has not been removed but a ligature had been tied distal to Hartmann's pouch.

Comment In view of these radiological appearances the T tube was removed and a further effort made to clear the duct. Small pieces of debris were obtained and after resiting the T tube a further X-ray (Fig. 9.4) was taken.

Question What does Fig. 9.4 show.
Answer
1 The normal beak-like ending of the common bile duct (1).
2 A possible false passage with extravasation of dye into the peripancreatic areolar tissue (2).

Comment Despite the absence of any flow of dye into the duodenum the operator (FGS) felt a satisfactory result had been achieved. The gall bladder was removed in the normal retrograde fashion and the

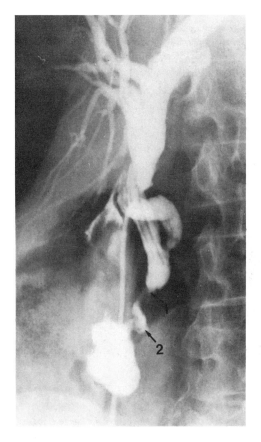

9.4

wound closed with catgut, a suction drain having been placed in the gall bladder bed.

Question A cholangiogram was performed on the 10th post-operative day. This is shown in Fig. 9.5. What does this demonstrate.

Answer

    1 The ampullary area with free flow of the contrast medium into the duodenum and the commencement of the pancreatic duct.

    2 Too long a cystic duct.

    3 A periVaterian diverticulum of the duodenum.

Question By what other techniques can calculi be removed from the common bile duct at the time of operation.

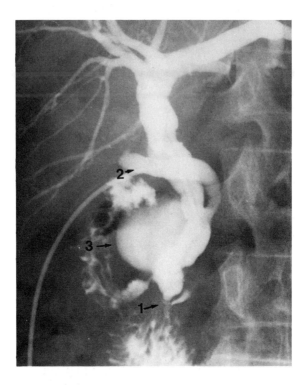

9.5

Answer

1 By transduodenal sphincteroplasty. This operation is performed by threading an umbilical catheter from the cystic duct, through the common bile duct and into the duodenum. The site of the ampulla of Vater is thus identified and the duodenum having been first mobilized, is opened.

A grooved Brodie's probe is then inserted into the open end of the umbilical catheter, tied in place and 'railroaded' in retrograde fashion through the ampulla into the common bile duct. Using right angled arteriotomy scissors the lower end of the common bile duct is laid open along the line of the fistula director for a variable distance after which the mucosa of the duodenum is sutured to the mucosa of the common bile duct. Contained calculi will then either extrude into the duodenum or can be removed by either DesJardin forceps or the method described below. The aim of sphincteroplasty is to produce a terminal end to side choledochoduodenostomy with a stoma equal in diameter to that of the largest part of the supraduodenal common bile duct. Once this has been achieved the opening is permanent and non-contractile since the entire sphincter mechanism is destroyed.

This procedure is associated with a mortality rate of approximately one per cent and a morbidity of approximately five per cent, transient pancreatitis, duodenal leakage and wound infection being the chief cause of concern.

2 By passing a Fogarty catheter through a choledochotomy into the duodenum and withdrawing it with the balloon distended. If the catheter has passed the ampulla and the balloon is then distended it will, on withdrawal, naturally impact first at the ampulla. At this point pressure is released and the catheter is withdrawn a few millimetres after which the balloon is again distended and withdrawn along the duct. This process can also be performed in a retrograde fashion. Figure 9.6 is an operative cholangiogram showing a number of calculi in the common bile duct together with a single calculus

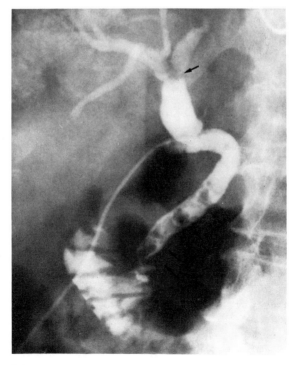

9.6

situated at the junction of the hepatic ducts which were successfully removed by this technique.

The potential complications of this manoeuvre are:

(a) intrahepatic rupture causing the development of 'bile lakes'.

(b) extrahepatic perforation.

(c) bleeding.

Comment Assuming a flexible cholodochoscope is available the complete clearance of the common bile duct can be ascertained visually. If such an instrument is not available and a transduodenal sphincteroplasty has not been performed the surgeon must rely on his own judgement having counted the number of calculi he expects to retrieve from the common duct or better perform a further operative cholangiogram before closing the common bile duct or inserting a T tube.

This patient made an uninterrupted recovery and the patient left hospital on the 12th post-operative day.

Question What is the accepted figure for retained calculi following supraduodenal exploration of the common bile duct.

Answer Three per cent even when meticulous technique is used.

Question Supposing a cholangiogram performed on the 10th post-operative day shows a retained stone in the common duct, what measures can be adopted.

Answer

1   A conservative approach. Clamp the T-tube and if the patient complains of neither pain nor jaundice pull out the T-tube and await events. This is a particularly acceptable method in the elderly, particularly if the calculus is less than 5 mm in diameter.

2   Percutaneous stone extraction. The T-tube is left *in situ* for a period of four to six weeks so that fibrosis can occur in the wall of the tract after which under fluoroscopic control an attempt is made to extract the stone using either:

(a) Desjardin forceps.

(b) A Dormia basket. This can be passed down the tract itself or better still, passed beyond the stone by using a steerable catheter with an external diameter of 4.3 mm (13 F).

(c) Yamakawe described removing the stones by means of a flexible choledochoscope, a technique requiring a tract able to take a 18 F instrument.

3   Perform an endoscopic sphincterotomy.

Question What complications may follow endoscopic sphincterotomy.

Answer Complications occur in between five and eight per cent of patients. They include:

1 Bleeding.
2 Pancreatitis.
3 Cholangitis.
4 Retroperitoneal perforation.

Question What is the success rate using any one of the above techniques.

Answer Those expert in the use of such techniques, claim about 95 per cent.

10

A female, 61 years of age, was admitted as an acute complaining of recurrent attacks of severe right-sided upper abdominal pain. On the day of admission the pain had not been relieved by an injection given by her own doctor. Each attack had followed a similar pattern; a feeling of unease in the upper abdomen after which constant pain had developed in the right subcostal region. During each attack she had been unable to find relief by altering her posture. There had been no radiation of pain to the back. At each attack she had had severe vomiting.

Previous history

1 At the age of 35 following the birth of her only child she had developed pain and swelling of the left leg.

2 At the age of 50 she had complained of paraesthesia and coldness of the left hand together with pain in the forearm whilst performing her housework.

3 At the age of 56 she had developed severe thirst and loss of weight. Investigation revealed diabetes which was controlled by diet together with oral hypoglycaemic agents.

4 Three years prior to this present admission she had complained of similar pain and had been investigated. A cholecystogram had shown no evidence of biliary calculi but a barium swallow had shown the presence of a hiatus hernia.

Physical examination Examination of the respiratory system revealed nothing of note except for a left thoracotomy scar along the line of the fourth rib. Examination of the upper limbs revealed no muscle wasting but an absent left radial pulse. Examination of the legs showed no swelling or ulceration but some scattered varicose veins of equal severity on both sides.

Question What diagnosis does this history suggest.

Answer Intermittent attacks of biliary colic due to gall-stones, this despite the negative investigation some three years previously.

Question In a patient suffering from severe pain at the time of examination what physical signs associated with biliary colic may be present.

Answer

1 Murphy's sign; pain on inspiration during gentle palpation of the right subcostal region.

2 Boas's sign; a localized area of cutaneous hyperaesthesia, elicited by scratching the skin with a fine needle over the area of the tip of the right shoulder blade.

Question What percentage of gall-stones are radio-opaque.

Answer Ten per cent.

Question Can a false negative result occur using oral cholecystography.

Answer Yes, but rarely. Failure to visualize non-opaque calculi in the absence of jaundice is usually due to one of the following causes:

1 The cystic duct is blocked by a calculus thus preventing the ingress of dye into the gall bladder.

2 If the mucosa of the gall bladder has been destroyed by prior attacks of inflammation the dye, normally solu-biloptin (Idopace) will not be concentrated and, therefore, no shadow will appear.

3 Very occasionally the contrast medium itself conceals contained calculi.

Question In view of the negative cholecystogram three years previously what investigation would you order.

Answer Ultrasonography of the biliary region. This investigation is highly specific but requires the contained calculi to be at least 3 mm in diameter before they can be identified as shadowing opacities which move within the gall bladder. It is especially valuable in the jaundiced patient (see Viva 9) and in the pregnant female.

Comment In this patient ultrasonography revealed multiple large calculi within the gall bladder.

Question What advice would you give.

Answer In this patient in view of the relatively short history, her previous and present medical history and the presence of non-opaque stones it would be reasonable to advise a conservative regime. She could be given a supply of analgesics to control the pain if it recurred and in addition an attempt could be made to dissolve the radiolucent calculi.

Question What drugs may produce dissolution of gall-stones.

Answer

1 Chenodeoxycholic acid, a bile salt, which acts by reducing the hepatic synthesis and biliary secretion of cholesterol. The normal dose is between 14 and 20 mg/kg of body weight daily, the larger dose being administered to obese patients. Calculi should be less than 15 mm in diameter, radiolucent and the gall bladder must be functioning. It may take several months before complete dissolution has occurred. Progress can be checked by ultrasonography at six monthly intervals. Small stones less than 5 mm in diameter may show signs of dissolution within a few months whereas larger stones may require continuous therapy for a period of several months.

2 Ursodeoxycholic acid. This drug also acts by decreasing the

secretion of cholesterol by the liver, normally administered in a dose of 450–600 mg daily in two divided doses. It is said to produce more rapid dissolution without inducing diarrhoea.

Question Is either drug effective in the treatment of pure pigment stones.

Answer No.

Question What percentage of stones can be expected to dissolve.

Answer Approximately 60 per cent.

Question What percentage recur after ceasing treatment.

Answer Approximately 30 per cent will have recurred within one year. To prevent this the suggestion has been made that a low dose should be continued.

Question Are any marked side effects associated with the administration of these drugs.

Answer Diarrhoea.

Question What drug could be used to control the pain?

Answer Pethidine, in a dose appropriate to the degree of pain.

Comment This patient stated that the pain was so severe that she preferred to undergo surgery. In view of this decision by the patient consideration must now be given to two other important aspects in her previous medical history:

1 The presence of forearm pain and the absent left radial pulse.
2 The post-partum history of pain and swelling in the left leg.

Question What significance do you attach to the left thorocotomy scar and the history preceding it?

Answer It suggests that the patient was suffering from atherosclerotic obstruction of the left subclavian artery.

Question What other additional symptoms in the affected upper limb might have been present.

Answer
1 Raynaud's phenomenon.
2 Subclavian steel syndrome.

Question What is the subclavian steel syndrome.

Answer It consists of attacks of transient cerebral ischaemia caused by reversal of the normal cephalic flow of blood in the vertebral arteries. The caudal flow of blood in the vertebral arteries provides the upper limb of blood from which it is deprived by blockage of the subclavian artery, the block normally occurring at its origin. This syndrome is rare in the absence of associated narrowing of the internal carotid artery due to the excellent intracranial circulation.

Question Is subclavian endarterectomy followed by good results.

Answer Very infrequently. In this patient the radial pulse, present immediately following operation was found to be absent within one month although the patient did admit to some symptomatic improvement. Ten years later the pulse remains absent and the patient continues to complain of pain in the hand during exercise.

Comment Following her thoracotomy the patient had considerable post-thoracotomy pain. This was so constant and severe that it was treated by phenol injection of three thoracic sensory nerves, segments 3, 4 and 5 without any appreciable improvement. Some three years later, however, an epidural injection of 5 ml of 0.5 per cent Marcain mixed with 40 mg of Depo-Medrone produced rapid and permanent pain relief.

Question Assuming that the post-partum pain and swelling of the left leg was due to a deep vein thrombosis, would prophylactic anti-coagulant therapy be advisable in this patient.
Answer Yes.

Comment In this patient heparin sodium was given. This is made up in disposable syringes with the needle attached, 5000 units in 0.2 ml.

Question How is the heparin administered and in what dose regime.
Answer Subcutaneously into the abdominal fat. Many alternative regimes have been described. The one used in this patient was 5000 units two hours prior to operation followed by 5000 units eight hourly for a period of five days. Whether this regime is more effective than others which have been described has never been the subject of a large controlled trial.

Comment A routine cholecystectomy was performed. On Day two, the patient complained of pain in the right side of the abdomen, physical examination revealing tenderness in this area.
Between Days 5 and 10 an intermittent temperature was present. On the 10th day partial dehiscence of the upper part of the wound occurred. However, the temperature remained elevated and oral hypoglycaemic agents failed to control the diabetes.

Question What does this suggest.
Answer The presence of an infected haematoma in Rutherford Morrison's pouch, i.e. the right subhepatic space.
Question Would this be associated with radiological changes on a plain X-ray of the chest.
Answer No. Only an inflammatory lesion of the right or left suprahepatic

spaces is associated with radiological changes in the chest, the commonest of which are elevation of the diaphragm, collapse/consolidation and an associated pleural effusion.

Question How can the presence of a subhepatic collection be confirmed.

Answer When the collection is large and of moderate duration a mass becomes palpable below the right costal margin. Smaller collections can be identified by ultrasonography. It is also possible under ultrasonic guidance to site a drain into the collection and thus avoid further surgical interference.

Question How would you control the diabetes.

Answer By substituting Atrapid in whatever dose is appropriate for the oral hypoglycaemic agent.

Comment On Day 20 after having apparently settled, the patient developed pain in the left calf, which although not swollen was tender on pressure.

Question In view of the previous history what is the most probable diagnosis.

Answer A left-sided deep vein thrombosis.

Question What is the most accurate method of confirming this diagnosis and assessing the extent of the lesion.

Answer By venography. This revealed an extensive clot in the deep veins of the calf and the femoral vein.

Question What treatment would you prescribe.

Answer Anticoagulant therapy. This was established using an intravenous line and administering 40000 units of heparin within 24 hours and thereafter 20000 units daily. The indirect anticoagulant warfarin BP 5–10 mg daily was also commenced within 24 hours, the aim being to produce an activated partial thromboplastin time (APTT) between 1.5 and twice normal.

Comment Despite anticoagulation on Day 21 the patient developed a cold blue painful left foot. Examination revealed absent left popliteal and posterior tibial pulses.

Question What are the possible causes.

Answer The differential diagnosis includes:

  1   An arterial embolus lodging at the origin of the profunda femoris artery. The absence of valvular heart disease, a recent myocardial infarct or an aortic aneurysm make this diagnosis unlikely.

  2   Arterial spasm associated with spread of the venous thrombus is

unlikely because venous thrombosis and arterial spasm, usually occur concurrently.

3 Thrombosis of the superficial femoral artery in the region of the adductor hiatus or haemorrhage beneath an atheromatous plaque in this area. This represents a distinct possibility in view of her known past history of arterial disease.

Question What possible lines of treatment could be considered.

Answer

1 Conclude that the arterial block had been present for some time and do nothing other than continuing the heparin regime already begun.

2 Consider localizing the site of the block by angiography and then giving a localized intra-arterial injection of streptokinase.

3 Discontinue heparin, reverse the prothrombin time, locate the exact site of obstruction and possibly perform some form of reconstructed arterial surgery or an angioplasty.

Comment After considerable discussion it was decided to do nothing other than continue the heparin schedule already started. Although the patient complained of intense pain in the calf especially on weight bearing, the limb continued to improve, as also did the patient herself, and the patient eventually left hospital 32 days after admission, anticoagulated on warfarin. Later investigation by Doppler ultrasound confirmed the presence of a block of the upper portion of the popliteal artery. However, when seen some six months later in the outpatient department the patient was not complaining of intermittent claudication or rest pain and physical examination, although revealing absent popliteal and posterior tibial pulses, showed no evidence of ischaemic changes in the foot. In view of this no active treatment was advised and when seen one year later her condition was unchanged.

11

A Caucasian female, aged 68, was admitted complaining of loss of 4 kg in weight over four weeks. One week prior to her initial attendance at the out-patient's department she had noted the onset of jaundice together with the passage of dark urine and pale stools, loss of appetite and indigestion. She also complained of slight upper abdominal pain but no pain in the back.

Previous medical history Little of importance, apart from the development of hypertension some 10 years previously for which she was receiving methyldopa (Aldomet, Merck, Sharp and Dohme) 250 mg daily and frusemide BP 40 mg daily.

Physical examination Inspection revealed an obviously jaundiced woman.

Cardiovascular system	BP 140/90 mmHg. JVP, −ve.
Respiratory system	No abnormality detected.
Abdominal examination	Liver palpable below costal margin, edge smooth, slightly tender. No other physical signs. Rectal examination, no abnormality palpated, pale stools on glove.

Question What are the chief adverse effects associated with methyldopa.

Answer Drowsiness, nightmares, nausea and dryness of the mouth.

Question What are the absolute contraindications to its use as an antihypertensive agent.

Answer Impaired renal or hepatic function.

Question What are the chief adverse effects of frusemide.

Answer Fluid and electrolyte imbalance.

Question Does the history suggest a diagnosis.

Answer Yes. A carcinoma of the head of the pancreas.

Question What physical sign is absent which would have made this diagnosis almost a clinical certainty.

Answer A palpable gall bladder.

Question What is Courvoisier's law.

Answer A palpable gall bladder in the presence of jaundice indicates that the jaundice is unlikely to be due to gall-stones.

Question What are the chief exceptions to this law.

Answer

1 In patients suffering from cholelithiasis the neck of the gall bladder may have become obstructed with the development of a mucocele of the gall bladder.

2   In a patient suffering from malignant obstructive jaundice, if the obstruction lies in the porta hepatis, as in malignant lymphadenopathy secondary to a cancer of the stomach the gall bladder cannot possibly dilate.

3   If the patient has suffered repeated attacks of cholecystitis the gall bladder will be fibrosed and shrunken and cannot, therefore, distend.

Question What are the chief biochemical changes you would expect to find in this patient.

Answer Elevation of:

1   serum bilirubin, normal value 16 μmol/l. (0.8 mg/100 ml).

2   alkaline phosphatase, normal value 3–13 King Armstrong units.

3   Only moderate elevation of the aminotransferases, normal value 11–35 IU/l.

Comment In this patient the following results were obtained:

1   Serum bilirubin 210 μmol/l.

2   Alkaline phosphatase 106 King Armstrong units.

3   Aminotransferases 50 IU/l.

Over the subsequent days during which pre-operative investigations were being carried out the serum bilirubin rose to 660 μmol/l.

Question Does the bilirubin continue to rise regardless of the length and severity of the obstruction.

Answer No. Because the greater part of the bilirubin is conjugated with glucuronic acid which is water soluble. Therefore, some is excreted in the urine hence its dark colour and after some weeks a balance occurs between its rate of production and excretion.

Question What haematological examination would you request.

Answer Prothrombin time.

Question Why.

Answer The prothrombin time may be prolonged because of failure to absorb the fat soluble Vitamin K.

Question What other factor is fat soluble and, therefore, not absorbed.

Answer Factor VII.

Question What clinical manifestation of Vitamin K deficiency may be present.

Answer Ready or spontaneous bruising and with a severe deficiency a tendency to excessive bleeding following injury.

Question If the prothrombin time is prolonged how would you correct it.

Answer By the intramuscular injection of Vitamin K_1, phytomenadione, 25 mg daily. The daily requirement in obstructive jaundice is between 100–500 ng/kg body weight.

Question Why is Vitamin K essential.

Answer Without adequate availability of Vitamin K, prothrombin, factors VII, IX and X are not generated in the liver.

Question What radiological investigations are necessary to make a diagnosis.

Answer

1   Abdominal ultrasound.
2   Percutaneous transhepatic cholangiography.

Comment The results of these investigations are shown in Figs 11.1 and 11.2.

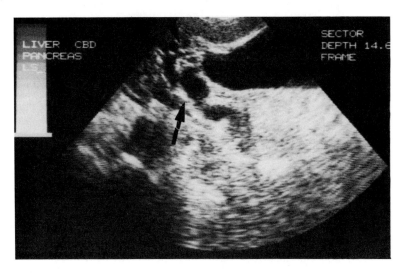

11.1

Question What do these show.

Answer The most important findings on ultrasonography are (Fig. 11.1):

1   The gall bladder is distended and contains no calculi.
2   The intrahepatic, common hepatic and common bile ducts are dilated as also is the pancreatic duct.
3   A small, soft tumour mass was identified at the lower end of the common duct within the head of the pancreas.

The percutaneous transhepatic cholangiogram (Fig. 11.2) shows a tapered neoplastic type of stricture at the lower end of the common bile duct which is causing complete obstruction and dilatation of the biliary system above it.

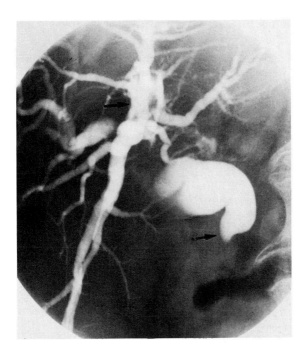

11.2

Comment These results confirm that we are dealing with a case of obstructive jaundice due to malignant obstruction of the lower end of the common bile duct caused by a small pancreatic neoplasm.

Question What methods of treatment are available.
Answer
    1 Palliative treatment.
    2 Radical treatment.
Question What methods of palliative treatment are available.
Answer
    1 Open operation followed by cholecystojejunostomy or cholecystoduodenostomy. Although both operations represent very simple technical exercises very high mortality rates have been reported in the literature following these operations varying between 15 and 25 per cent.
    2 An internally placed catheter. Three variations of this technique have been described in patients in whom radiological techniques assess the pancreatic neoplasm as being inoperable:

(a) an internally placed catheter with an open end on the surface which can be blocked.

(b) a permanent endoprosthesis using a 12 F polyethylene tube. The advantage of this technique is that the patient is relieved of the psychological trauma associated with a permanent externally draining catheter. The disadvantages are:

(i) the loss of access for tubal irrigation.

(ii) blockage entails replacement.

(iii) one cannot perform repetitive cholangiograms to assess the progress of the disease.

(c) the placement of a prosthesis by means of an endoscope, a method first described by Sochendra and others in 1979. This method, if available, is particularly applicable in frail patients. A high rate of initial technical success can be achieved but there is a high level of readmission for local complications.

All these various methods of palliation by conservative means are acceptable unless the duodenum is also obstructed or becoming obstructed.

Question Using a small diameter catheter, bile may fail to drain into the duodenum for some five to six days. Why is this.

Answer Because of the viscosity of the bile. Unlike water, bile is a Bingham plastic. Therefore it does not flow until a threshold driving pressure has been reached, this threshold depending on its viscosity.

Question What is the normal pressure differential between the intrahepatic bile ducts and the duodenum.

Answer 30–35 cm to 10–15 cm of water.

Question What radiological signs indicate that a pancreatic neoplasm is inoperable.

Answer 'Encasement' of the branches of the coeliac axis artery and visible invasion as opposed to displacement of the portal vein on portal venography. A barium meal showing distortion and rigidity of the duodenal mucosa.

Question What percentage of pancreatic neoplasms are surgically resectable at the time of clinical presentation.

Answer Only some 10–15 per cent.

Question What is the five year survival in patients treated by 'curative' resection.

Answer Fifteen per cent.

Question What is the mean survival time following palliative surgery.

Answer Six months.

Question What is the peri-operative mortality of radical resection.

Answer Figures between 10 and 60 per cent are quoted.

Question Prior to surgical exploration what other investigations might help to determine the operability or otherwise of a tumour in the head of the pancreas.

Answer If available, a CAT scan. This may clearly show evidence not only of local invasion but also portal vein involvement and the presence of enlarged lymph nodes.

Question What, apart from 'surgical ineptitude' are the chief factors influencing the mortality following operations to relieve obstructive jaundice.

Answer Three factors appear to be of importance:

1 Haemocrit, if less than 30 per cent.
2 A plasma bilirubin in excess of 200 µmol/l.
3 The presence of malignancy as a cause for the jaundice.

Comment The abdomen was explored via an upper transverse, abdominal incision and a total pancreatectomy performed. Although enlarged lymph nodes were present in the peripancreatic tissues these were later found on microscopic examination to be free of malignancy. The tumour itself proved to be a well differentiated adenocarcinoma of the pancreas with perineural invasion. It measured 1.2 cm in diameter. The body and tail of the pancreas showed the classical histological changes of chronic pancreatitis.

Question What is the advantage of total pancreatectomy compared to Whipple's operation.

Answer The surgeon avoids the dangers associated with the difficult anastomosis between the pancreatic duct and the jejunum, leakage from this anastomosis being the chief cause of peri-operative morbidity and mortality.

Question What, if any, are the disadvantages associated with total pancreatectomy.

Answer

1 The patient becomes diabetic.
2 Pancreatic exocrine deficiency inevitably occurs.
3 The spleen is removed resulting in an increased susceptibility to infection.

Comment In this patient a Roux-en-Y loop was fashioned and closed, it was then brought up through the mesocolon. An end to side choledochojejunostomy was performed after which, having removed the antrum, the stomach was anastomosed end to side to the Roux loop. Following operation the jaundice began to wane with great rapidity and by the 10th post-operative day, the total bilirubin had fallen to 36 µmols/l and the alkaline phosphatase to 24 KA units.

However, on the fifth post-operative day the nasogastric aspirate began to increase and frank blood was obtained, this despite the fact that the patient was already receiving ranitidine 50 mg bd intravenously. However, the Hb level was found to be normal and no transfusion, other than crystalloid was given.

On the following day a bile stained nasogastric aspirate of over 2 litres was obtained.

Question What does this suggest.

Answer A small gut obstruction distal to both the gastrojejunostomy and the choledochojejunostomy.

Question How could this diagnosis be confirmed.

Answer By barium studies. In this patient, however, only gastrografin studies were performed. These are notoriously unreliable because the medium is water soluble and all that was shown was that the medium passed rapidly into the jejunum.

The result of the gastrografin swallow is shown in Fig. 11.3. Although there is a suggestion that proximal small bowel obstruction is present, the upper arrow pointing to a somewhat distended portion

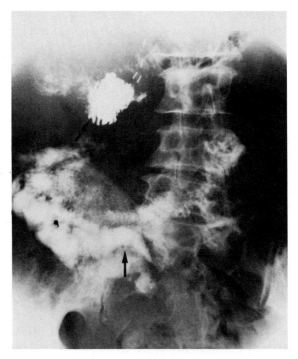

11.3

of bowel, the lower arrow shows that there was no hold up to the passage of contrast medium into the distal small bowel; a finding which totally 'disarmed' both the radiologist and the surgeon.

Comment In view of this radiological report and because the nasogastric aspirate rapidly diminished over the succeeding two days no further action was taken and on the 12th post-operative day the nasogastric tube was removed. On the 15th day the temperature rose to 38.6°C and the patient complained of feeling unwell. The abdomen was distended and a vomit of a few millimetres of bile-stained fluid occurred

Question What investigations would you order in view of the above.
Answer Blood culture. Plain X-ray of abdomen.

Comment The blood culture was negative. Two fluid levels were present on the abdominal radiograph but no grossly dilated loops were seen. The following day, there being no aspirate, the nasogastric tube was once again removed and small quantities of fluid by mouth were given. Three days later the patient was beginning to eat solid food and stabilization of the diabetic state began, the patient having until this time being maintained on intravenous insulin according to blood sugar levels.

She was finally discharged thirty-one days after operation on 10 units of Mixtard insulin in a morning and 6 units at 18.00 hours, together with three capsules of Pancrex to be taken with each meal, each capsule to be opened and sprinkled on the food to be eaten.
Question What is Pancrex.
Answer Pancrex (Paines and Byrne UK), pancreatin BP is a preparation of mammalian pancreas containing enzymes having protease, lipase and amylase activity. Each gram contains not less than 1400 BP units of protease activity, not less than 25000 units of lipase activity and not less than 30000 units of amylase activity. By providing three capsules with each meal approximately 1 g of pancreatin is being given.

Comment The patient was seen as an out-patient at monthly intervals following her discharge. One major difficulty was the control of her diabetes and various alterations to the insulin schedule were proposed. Six months after her initial surgery the following insulin regime was in use, Initard 24 units in the morning and 12 units in the afternoon. Five months following surgery her weight was steady and her bowels were open once a day. She was, however, complaining of flatulence.

Readmission Precisely seven months after surgery she was admitted complaining of:

1 General malaise of two months duration.

2 Abdominal pain of one month's duration. She described the pain in the following terms, band-like, intermittent and aggravated by movement.

3 Intermittent vomiting for one week, chiefly bile.

4 Loss of 14 kilos.

Physical examination This revealed a dehydrated woman whose skin turgor was greatly diminished.

Abdominal examination Inspection revealed slight distension above and to the right of the umbilicus.

A succession splash was present in the upper abdomen. Auscultation confirmed the presence of the splash but no excessive bowel sounds were present.

Question What is a working diagnosis.

Answer Subacute intestinal obstruction.

Question What steps are required.

Answer

1 Relieve vomiting by means of nasogastric suction.

2 Rehydrate the patient by means of intravenous therapy.

3 Confirm the diagnosis by means of a plain X-ray of the abdomen.

4 A fluid input and output chart.

5 Take blood for electrolyte and urea evaluation.

6 Begin intravenous insulin on a sliding scale.

7 Catheterize the patient so that the urine output can be accurately measured.

Comment All these steps were taken. On the day following admission, however, the patient's temperature rose to 38.3°C.

Question What investigation is required.

Answer A blood culture.

Comment This revealed both Gram positive and Gram negative organisms, later identified as *Escherichia coli, Klebsiella oxytoca* and *Clostridium* sp., sensitive to gentamicin, cephalosporin and metronidazole. The total nucleated cell count on this day was 21×10^9/l.

Question What does the pyrexia coupled with a positive blood culture indicate.

Answer The presence of septicaemia.

Question Can you explain how this patient has become septicaemic.

Answer A reasonable working hypothesis would be that obstruction to the jejunal loop distal to the choledochojejunostomy had led to an ascending cholangitis and hence because of unrelieved obstruction to septicaemia.

Comment On the second day following admission the abdomen was explored. The chief operative findings were:

1 normal small bowel distal to the level of the transverse mesocolon.

2 dilatation of the jejunum loop proximal to the level of the transverse mesocolon.

3 a dilated gastric remnant.

4 a white nodule approximately 2 cm in diameter in a subcapsular position on the right lobe of the liver.

5 the obstructing agent proved to be the transverse mesocolon, dissection in this area leading to an area of hard, adipose tissue in which fibrosis, possibly secondary to fat necrosis had occurred.

Question How would you relieve the situation.

Answer The simplest solution would be to perform a jejuno-jejunostomy anterior to the transverse colon thus by-passing the obstructing agent. This was performed.

Question In view of the septicaemia should this operation be 'covered' with antibiotics.

Answer Undoubtedly yes. In this case the three antibiotics to which the organisms found on blood culture were sensitive, were administered.

Comment On the first post-operative day the patient's general condition rapidly deteriorated.

Physical examination revealed the following:

1 Pulse rate: 120

2 Respiration rate: 40

3 Blood pressure: 130/60

A plain X-ray of the chest showed right sided basal consolidation.

Examination of the fluid balance charts revealed that the urine output had fallen to 10 ml/hour.

The hands and feet were cold and cyanotic and the patient was sweating profusely.

Question What has happened and what investigation might be helpful in management.

Answer It is reasonable to assume that the patient is suffering from septicaemic 'shock'.

Investigations

1 Blood Gases: PO_2 = 7.0 kPa
                PCO_2 = 3.6 kPa
                pH = 7.4
                HCO_3 = 17.0
                O_2 saturation = 86%

2 Electrolytes: Na = 131 mmol/l
                K = 4.1 mmol/l
                Cl = 98 mmol/l

Question What steps in the management of this patient would you take.

Answer

1 Insert a central venous pressure line: in this patient the CVP was −4 cm at the sternal angle.

2 Give the bed a 15–20° foot-tilt which increases filling of the right ventricle and, therefore, helps to improve cardiac output.

3 The administration of humidified oxygen.

4 Obviously the patient is 'hypovolaemic' from pooling of blood in the microcirculation and leakage of fluid, electrolytes and plasma from the same area. Two litres of normal saline with added potassium were given followed by two litres of plasma protein fraction. This raised the central venous pressure to above 3 cm, and the blood pressure to 130/80 mmHg and the urine output rose. This last was of great importance in view of a plasma urea of 10.6 mmol/l (N value = 2.5–7.1 mmol/l) and the fact that the patient had received gentamicin.

Question What deductions can we draw from the central venous pressure measurement.

Answer If the CVBP is high, a fact which may be obvious on clinical examination, the shock state is due to impaired cardiac function whereas if the CVP is low, below 2 cm of water, as measured from the sternal angle the shock state is due to inadequate cardiac filling and urgent attention must be given to restoring the circulatory blood volume.

Question What is the importance of adequate renal function in patients receiving gentamicin.

Answer Patients suffering from renal impairment are especially liable to develop vestibular damage and high tone deafness. Furthermore reversible nephrotoxicity together with acute renal failure may occur, particularly in patients who are concurrently receiving cephalosporin antibiotics.

Question How do you guard against such complications.

Answer

1 In patients in whom renal failure is suspected only one dose of gentamicin should be given.

2 Gentamicin levels in the plasma should be estimated; concentrations above 10–12 μg/ml carry a high risk of ototoxicity.

3 Alter the antibiotic regime.

Comment Ampicillin was substituted for cephradine.

Question What important complication of septic shock other than renal failure may occur.

Answer Disseminated intravascular coagulation.

Question What single test would confirm that this process was occurring.

Answer The presence of fibrinogen degradation products in the circulation.

Comment In this patient, FDP values rose as high as 64 μg/l but the prothrombin time although abnormal, rising to 18/13 seconds, never reached dangerous levels and the plasma fibrinogen levels never fell below 2.3 g/l (N value = 3.49 g/l). These results show that some defibrination was occurring but that the condition was subclinical. On the following day the patient was considerably improved. The urine output had risen to 100 ml/h, the temperature had fallen from 38 to 36.5°C, the pulse rate to 80 per minute but the blood pressure still remained low (110/60 mmHg).

Question Had the blood pressure failed to rise despite the correction of the 'hypovolaemia' what deduction would you make.

Answer That cardiac function must be impaired.

Question What might you have done.

Answer In these circumstances the administration of dopamine by continuous intravenous infusion might produce benefit.

Question What is dopamine.

Answer A sympathomimetic agent with direct effects on beta-adrenergic receptors and indirect effects on alpha-adrenergic receptors. In the body it is a precursor of noradrenaline. It differs, however, from adrenaline and noradrenaline in dilating the renal and mesenteric blood vessels and increasing urine output. In addition the inotropic action of dopamine on the heart is associated with less cardiac-accelerating effect than isoprenaline. This dual action of dopamine is extremely valuable in the treatment of shock.

The chief indication for the use of dopamine is in the treatment of 'shock' failing to respond to adequate restoration of the circulating blood volume.

Question What dose would you use.

Answer An initial dose of 2–5 μg/kg body weight/min gradually increasing to 5–10 μg/kg per min according to the patient's response as measured by the blood pressure and urine output. High doses in the region of 50 μg/kg per min have been used.

Question What complication must be avoided.

Answer Tissue necrosis by using a vein high in the arm and inserting a long, fine catheter.

Comment On the following day although the patient's general condition appeared much improved her temperature suddenly rose to 39°C, PR to 110 and the CVP fell to −5 cm. The blood pressure, however, remained stable. A rigor occurred.

Question What does this suggest.

Answer A further septicaemic episode.

Comment This episode was treated by the administration of human plasma protein fraction, the administration of four litres of humidified oxygen per minute and a change in the antibiotic regime to piperacillin 2 g every six hours, gentamicin 80 mg tds and metronidazole. The last drug was given intravenously in a five per cent solution, 100 ml every eight hours at a rate of 5 ml/min.

Question What is the advantage of substituting piperacillin for ampicillin.

Answer Piperacillin is considered to be more active *in vitro* than either ampicillin or carbenicillin against Gram negative organism.

Question What is the reason for administering metronidazole.

Answer Metronidazole is active against obligate anaerobic bacteria such as *Bacteroides* and *Fusobacterium* spp.

Comment On the following day the urine volume had fallen to 10 ml/h. The BP was 90/40, PR 110, the CVP −5 cm and the Tp. 39°C. The blood gases were as follows: PO_2, 7.3; pCO_2, 4.3; pH, 7.47; O_2 saturation 89%. The septicaemic episode had, therefore, continued. Examination revealed dullness to percussion at both bases with marked crepitations. The urine output was negligible and haematological examination revealed Hb 9.2. Platelets 11×10^9/l.

Question In the absence of any overt evidence of haemorrhage, what does the fall in the Hb level signify.

Answer Haemolysis must be occurring. That this was so was substantiated by the finding of a haemolytic streptococcus on a further blood culture.

Comment A further unit of blood was given followed by four units of plasma protein fraction and two litres of saline. The CVP then rose to +7 cm without any improvement in the urine output.

Question If the blood volume was restored without any significant rise in urine output, what would you do.

Answer Give frusemide. In this case after the administration of 40 mg of frusemide the urine output rose to acceptable levels and continued thereafter to cause no problems.

Question What is the interval between the time of administration of frusemide and its effect.

Answer Following intravenous administration, frusemide produces its diuretic effect in approximately five minutes, the effect lasting about two hours.

Question Is a platelet count of $11 \times 10^9/l$ a cause for concern.

Answer Certainly. At this level any additional trauma is almost certain to be followed by haemorrhage, indeed bleeding may occur spontaneously at this platelet level.

Question Would you, therefore, give a platelet transfusion.

Answer No.

Question Why.

Answer Because platelets have a very short life (2–3 days) and the patient is not bleeding. Many patients receiving repeated platelet transfusions from random donors become refractory to treatment.

12

A Caucasian male aged 74 years was admitted complaining of severe epigastric pain of sudden onset radiating to the back. Since the onset of the pain some seven hours previously he had vomited on two occasions. He gave no history of alcohol abuse and indeed stated that he was teetotal.

His previous medical history was extensive:

1   At 50 years of age he had developed pain in the neck radiating into the right shoulder area following a golf match.

2   At 61 years of age he had developed increasing deafness. Examination had shown bilateral central perforations of the tympanic membranes.

3   At 62 years of age he had complained of increasing abdominal dyspepsia. A barium meal at this time had demonstrated a duodenal ulcer. Over the intervening years this had been treated, when symptomatic, first with antacids and later with H_2 antagonists.

4   At 65 years of age he had collapsed in the lavatory. Following admission to hospital he confessed to exertional dyspnoea over several years. No physical abnormality was discovered except for the presence of generalized rhonchi in both lung fields. His BP was 140/70 mmHg.

5   At 67 years of age he had developed angina pectoris, adequately controlled by the sublingual glyceryl trinitrate tablets when necessary. At the time of admission the patient was rolling around the bed in pain and was extremely reluctant to be examined. However, his PR was 60/min and his BP 170/120 mmHg. When he at last consented to be examined he was found to be tender over the whole of his abdomen.

Question Discuss the cause of his neck pain.

Answer A first episode of neck pain at the age of 50 might suggest that he may have suffered a simple 'sprain' of the neck caused by some sudden movement during the course of his golf match. Normally a simple sprain causes stiffness of the neck, symmetrical restriction of neck movement and diffuse tenderness on palpation with no other objective physical signs. These symptoms are rapidly relieved by wearing a cervical collar, particularly when in bed. In a younger individual one would expect X-rays of the cervical spine to show no evidence of any abnormality but at 50 years of age cervical spondylosis may be present.

Question What is cervical spondylosis.

Answer Cervical spondylosis is a term now in common use. However, a definition which satisfies orthopaedic surgeons, radiologists and pathologists is difficult to find. It is, however, generally accepted that it is a pathological condition of the cervical spine in which the most significant changes occur in the region of the facet joints, a change which can be demonstrated radiologically. The severity of these changes is related to age and whilst commonly asymptomatic, symptoms in the established disease, may be readily precipitated even by minor injury.

It was once considered that the initial pathological change giving rise to cervical spondylosis was degeneration of the cervical intervertebral discs, degeneration of these discs leading to stretching of the annulus fibrosus which if severe would be lifted from the margins of the vertebrae precipitating osteophyte formation, the osteophytes protruding not only into the spinal canal but also laterally into the intervertebral foraminae. As degeneration proceeded it was thought that the posterior spinal facet joints were placed under an increasing load with the result that degeneration of these joints was then precipitated leading to further osteophyte formation. This caused, because of its site, narrowing of the intervertebral canal from behind and nipping of the cervical nerve roots which in this part of the spinal cord run in an almost transverse manner from the cord through the intervertebral foraminae.

This theory is not supported, however, by the fact that degeneration of the facet joints is most marked at C_2, C_1 and C_3 whereas disc degeneration is most marked in the region of C_5, C_6 and C_7.

Question What are the commonest causes of central perforation of the tympanic membrane.

Answer

1 Infection of the middle ear, otitis media secondary to nasopharyngeal infection.

2 Compression, a force striking the external ear, e.g. a blow. A sudden increase in pressure in the external meatus by an explosion or the sudden inflow of water as in water skiing.

3 Instrumentation, usually accidental when cleaning the ears.

Comment The development of a duodenal ulcer at 62 years of age is important when considering the history on admission and the associated physical signs because the diagnosis of a perforated duodenal ulcer remains a possible cause of his symptoms until excluded.

Question Does a patient with a perforated bowel associated with generalized abdominal tenderness normally roll about.

Answer No, classically all patients suffering from peritoneal irritation remain still, not moving the abdominal wall so as not to irritate the inflamed peritoneum.

Question What other diagnosis would explain the history and physical signs.

Answer Acute pancreatitis. Note, a leaking aortic aneurysm could cause a very similar history but hypotension is commonly present immediately following the rupture. In this case the BP was actually higher than one recorded some years previously.

Question In view of the two most probable diagnoses what investigations would you order.

Answer Because of the patient's inability to remain still, straight X-rays of the abdomen which demand co-operation on the part of the patient would be practically useless. Therefore reliance must be placed on biochemical investigation.

Question Assuming that the patient was able to co-operate what radiological physical signs might be seen in: (a) a perforated peptic ulcer; (b) acute pancreatitis.

Answer (a) Using supine and erect films gas, i.e. a pneumoperitoneum will be found in approximately 60 per cent of patients. Since fluid is also present in the abdomen a fluid level may also be identified at the site of the pneumoperitoneum. In the erect film a small quantity of air causes a sickle-shaped translucency between the diaphragm above and the liver below.

(b) The commonest radiological physical sign is the presence of a single dilated segment of small bowel in the upper abdomen, the 'sentinel' loop. In severe cases of acute pancreatitis generalized distension of intestinal loops may be seen. Because of the relationship between gall-stones and acute pancreatitis the former may be visible on a plain X-ray.

Comment The following haematological and biochemical results were obtained:

Full blood count.	Total nucleated cell count	$13.8 \times 10^{12}/l$
	Hg	15.2 g/dl
	Platelet count	$455 \times 10^{a}/l$
	Sodium	13.8 mmol/l
	Potassium	3.9 mmol/l
	Calcium	2.23 mmol/l
	Urea	4.6 mmol/l

110

Serum amylase	1940 Somogyi units
Blood glucose	10.20 mmol/l
Total bilirubin	14 μ/mmol/l
Total protein	75 g/l

Question What deduction do you draw from these results.

Answer The serum amylase, normally 80–150 Somogyi units is grossly elevated supporting the diagnosis of acute pancreatitis.

Question Is the serum amylase raised in any other conditions.

Answer Yes. A raised serum amylase may be found in patients suffering from perforated peptic ulceration, acute cholecystitis, strangulation of the small bowel and also in terminal renal failure. However, in perforated peptic ulceration, for example, the serum amylase is within normal limits in over 80 per cent of patients and rarely exceeds 600 units in the remainder.

Question What other results, if any, are abnormal.

Answer

1   The fasting blood sugar, value 10.20 mmol/l (223 mg per cent) is well above the normal range of 2.5–4.7 mmol/l (65–105 mg per cent). This abnormal result is associated with temporary failure of the islet cells due to the inflammation surrounding them.

2   The serum calcium, value 2.23 mmol/l (9.25 mg per cent) is slightly below the normally accepted values of 2.25–2.60 mmol/l (9.50–10.25 mg per cent). The total serum calcium concentration falls in acute pancreatitis because calcium combines with the fatty acids formed from the hydrolysis of fat. These combine with the ionic calcium component of the plasma. The severity of the fall has been related to prognosis, a reduction of 30 per cent or more is regarded as extremely serious.

Question What are the commonest aetiological factors in acute pancreatitis.

Answer

1   Gall-stones.

2   Alcoholism.

These are the two commonest causes of acute pancreatitis and comprise the bulk of all reported series. However, their relative importance varies. For example, in Great Britain alcohol is more often associated with acute pancreatitis in Scotland, 20–25 per cent, than in England, 10 per cent. Alcohol is also a relatively common factor in North America and France.

Question What other less common causes have been identified.

Answer

1   Hyperparathyroidism.

111

2 Hyperlipidaemia.

3 Carcinoma of the ampulla or head of pancreas.

4 Mumps, in which pancreatitis tends to complicate the disease more commonly in teenagers and young adults rather than children in whom the disease is commonest.

5 Post-operative pancreatitis:

(a) following a Polya (Billroth II) type of gastrectomy.

(b) endoscopic ampullary sphincterotomy.

(c) transduodenal sphincterotomy for the treatment of choledocholithiasis.

6 Drugs: long continued treatment with high doses of steroids.

Question How would you treat this particular patient in view of the data already obtained.

Answer

1 By the administration of intravenous fluids. Depending on the severity of the disease simple crystalloid solutions may be sufficient. In more severe disease colloids may be required and at some stage a blood transfusion may be necessary.

2 Relieve pain with opiates.

Question Does nasogastric suction play any part in treatment.

Answer It is doubtful whether continuous nasogastric suction affects the course of the disease but by reducing vomiting it may diminish the discomfort suffered by the patient.

Question What other biochemical tests are of value in determining the severity of the disease or discriminating between the two most common causes, i.e. gall-stones or alcohol.

Answer

1 Plasma aspartate aminotransferase (AST). The circulating level of this enzyme is a sensitive indicator of hepatocyte disruption. A rise in AST, cut off point 60 iu/l, has been recorded in over 80 per cent of patients suffering from pancreatitis associated with gall-stones. An elevation of this enzyme is consistent with the concept that transient ampullary obstruction is associated with the development of pancreatitis.

2 γ-glutamyl transpeptidase, normal values in the male 6–28 iu/l, in the female 4–18 iu/l. Elevation of this enzyme above base levels suggests alcoholic pancreatitis probably due to microsomal enzyme induction by alcohol.

3 Plasma alanine aminotransferase, elevation of this enzyme has been related by some observers but not by others to the severity of the disease.

4 C reactive protein. An elevation of CRP is a non specific response to tissue injury, a rapid response normally occurs to changes in the intensity of the inflammatory stimulus. Levels above 100 mg/l at the end of the first week of the disease can be correlated with an increased risk of developing pancreatic collections.

5 Lactic dehydrogenase, LDH. Normal value, 150 iu/l is also an index of hepato-cellular injury.

Question What are Ranson's criteria of severity.

Answer Ranson in 1976 considered that eleven objective signs correlate with prognosis. On admission:

1 Age over 55 years.
2 WBC over 16×10^{12}/l.
3 Blood glucose in excess of 9.5 mmol/l, 200 mg per cent.
4 Serum lactic dehydrogenase above 350 iu/l.
5 Plasma aspartate aminotransferase over 250 units per cent.

During the initial 24 hours:

6 A decrease in the haematocrit of over 10 per cent.
7 A rise in blood urea.
8 Serum calcium falling below 1.9 mmol/l (8 mg per cent).
9 Arterial O_2 tension falling below 7.5 kPa (60 mmHg).
10 Base deficit of over 4 mmol/l (4 mEq/l).
11 Estimated sequestration of fluid over 6 l.

He noted in his series of 162 patients suffering from acute pancreatitis that in the presence of only two of these factors there were no deaths, thereafter the mortality progressively increased. Thus in the presence of six positive indicators 63 per cent of the patients died.

Imrie after studying 161 patients considered that an attack of pancreatitis could be considered severe if within 48 hours of admission three or more of the following nine factors were present:

1 WBC in excess of 15×10^{12}/l.
2 Serum calcium less than 2 mmol/l (8.4 mg per cent).
3 Serum albumin less than 32 g/l.
4 PaO_2 less than 7.5 kPa (60 mmHg).
5 LDH above 600 iu/l.
6 Transaminase enzymes in excess of 1000 iu/l.
7 Plasma glucose in excess of 10 mmol/l.
8 No response to intravenous fluids.
9 Age if greater than 55 years.

Question Is this patient, therefore, suffering from a severe attack of pancreatitis.

Answer No. Only two factors are present in both classifications, i.e. age over 55. Blood sugar in excess of 10 mmol/l.

Comment It would, therefore, be reasonable to expect this patient to recover from this attack without developing any serious life threatening complications.

On the day following admission his serum amylase had fallen to 1110 Somoygi units. However, he had become slightly jaundiced; total bilirubin 26 μmol/l (normal range 3–15 μmol/l), his total protein had fallen to 65 g/l (normal range 67–82 g/l) and the calcium level to 1.98 mmol/l. However, the glucose level had fallen to 6.20 mmol/l (normal range 3.3–5.6 mmol/l).

The fall in serum amylase, suggests that recovery is taking place but the falling serum calcium suggests that the saponification of neutral fat is continuing.

Question What invasive investigation has been used to determine the severity of pancreatitis.

Answer Peritoneal lavage. Using this technique, a severe attack, i.e. one which will have a complicated course possibly ending in death, is indicated by the presence of more than 10 ml of free peritoneal fluid at the initial tap or the withdrawal of brown coloured (prune juice) fluid following lavage.

Question What further biochemical investigation should be performed on this patient.

Answer Investigate the presence or absence of lipidaemia. This was done, the following results were obtained.

Triglycerides 1.08 mmol/l. Total cholesterol 3.6 mmol/l.

Appearance of the serum clear, chylomicron's absent.

Question Are these results within normal limits.

Answer Yes. The upper limit of triglycerides is 1.7 mmol/l and the total cholesterol over 49 years of age should be between 3.9–8 mmol/l.

Question Should the biliary system be investigated as the patient is now apparently recovering and co-operative.

Answer Yes.

Question What method would you use.

Answer Several methods are available:

1 Oral cholecystography is relatively inaccurate, visualization of the gall bladder occurring in only about 50 per cent of patients possibly due to oedema of the cystic duct in the acute phase blocking the ingress of dye into the gall bladder. In only 30–50 per cent of cases does this investigation help. Similar results occur with radionuclide biliary scanning using $N-N^1-2,6$-diethylphenyl carbamoxyl methyl iminodiacetic acid labelled with 3m Ci of $^{99}Tc^m$ which is administered intravenously. Visualization of the gall bladder and an absence of stones favours a diagnosis of alcohol induced pancreatitis.

Potentially the most satisfactory method of establishing the presence of cholithiasis is by the use of ultrasound which will not only give information about the gall bladder but will also indicate the size of the common bile duct and give some indication about the state of the pancreas.

Question What can you see on the ultrasound (Fig. 12.1) performed six days after the onset of his illness.

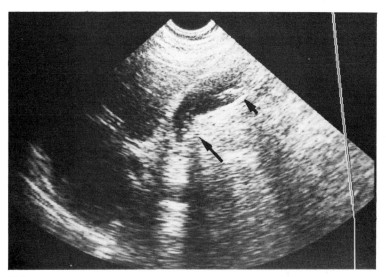

12.1

Answer Multiple stones in the gall bladder. The marked shadowing effect produced by biliary calculi is due to the attenuation of the beam during its passage through the stones.

Comment The patient was discharged on the following day with a diagnosis of mild acute pancreatitis secondary to biliary disease to return for routine cholecystectomy in three months.

Question Was this the correct decision.

Answer Probably not. In 1975 the first papers suggesting that cholecystectomy during an attack of acute pancreatitis caused by gall-stones was safe and effective. Following these papers others have appeared showing that regardless of the severity of the initial attack 56 per cent of patients awaiting elective cholecystectomy developed further symptoms. It has been suggested that an aggressive approach in pancreatitis due to cholelithiasis significantly lowers the mortality rate and that the mortality when an aggressive approach is used will be restricted to the elderly.

Comment Sixteen days after discharge the patient was readmitted complaining of severe upper abdominal pain. He insisted that he had been free of pain for only one day after discharge from hospital. In addition to severe pain he had repeatedly vomited especially at night and lost his appetite. Since his last admission he had lost four kilograms and appeared emaciated.

Examination at this time revealed no apparent anaemia, no cyanosis and no jaundice. His BP was 160/100. Chest examination revealed widespread inspiratory and expiratory crepitations. However, he was again uncooperative but he appeared to be tender across the whole of the upper abdomen.

The following biochemical results were obtained:

Serum amylase: 1480 Somogyi units

Serum calcium: 2.19 mmol/l

Blood sugar: 5.7 mmol/l

Serum albumin: 36 g/l

His blood gases breathing air were:

pCO_2 4.8 kPa (N 4.8–5.8)

pO_2 8 kPa (N > 8.6)

Actual HCO_3, 23 mmol/l (calculated 22.31)

O_2 saturation 92% (calculated 92–96)

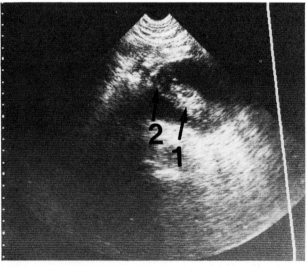

12.2

Question What investigations, other than biochemical data, would be of value in assessing his condition.

Answer Abdominal ultrasound.

Question What does the ultrasound examination show (Fig. 12.2).

Answer A swollen pancreas surrounded in the area of the body with an echo poor area compatible with the presence of a pseudocyst encircling the entire pancreas, diameter approximately 6 cm.

Comment Two days after his admission he was still distressed, complaining of severe abdominal pain, profuse vomiting and inability to eat.

Question In view of the continued inability to eat and the gross loss of weight found on this admission what treatment would you prescribe.

Answer Parenteral feeding. A central line was inserted after which a skin tunnel approximately 6 cm in length was made.

Question What would be a suitable regime.

Answer Freamine 1 l, 500 ml of 20 per cent glucose, 500 ml of Novoplex 1600 together with 500 ml of Intralipid on alternate days. In addition trace elements must be provided together with vitamins, the former are supplied as Addamel (KabiVitrum) and the latter as Solivito (KabiVitrum) with the addition of folic acid 10 mg and Vitamin B_{12} 15 mg once per week.

Comment Persistent pain continued and repeated pancreatic ultrasonography demonstrated that the pseudocyst was slowly enlarging (Fig. 12.3). Twelve days after admission a mass was palpable in the upper

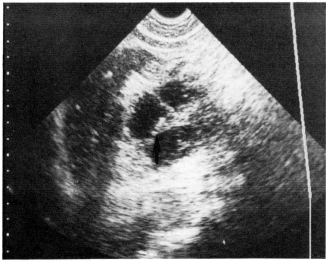

12.3

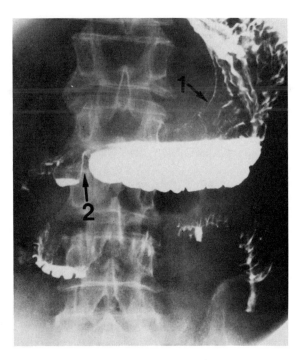

12.4

abdomen. A barium meal was performed (Fig. 12.4). This showed forward displacement of the stomach confirming the presence of a pseudocyst.

Question What action would you take.
Answer Laparotomy is indicated on the following grounds:
    1   the continuing severe pain,
    2   the persistent vomiting which suggests gastric outlet obstruction,
    3   the persistence and increasing diameter of the pancreatic pseudocyst.
Question What is a pancreatic pseudocyst.
Answer A collection of fluid and debris rich in pancreatic enzymes in the region of the pancreas or within the pancreatic parenchyma with no epithelial lining. An essential prerequisite to the development of such a cyst is disruption of the pancreatic ductal system.
Question What complications follow the development of a pseudocyst.
Answer Complications occur in approximately one-third of pancreatic pseudocysts. The common ones are:
    1   Obstruction to an adjacent organ, e.g. the duodenum or common bile duct.

2 Rupture into an adjacent organ, e.g. the stomach. This may be followed by severe haemorrhage, the left gastric artery being eroded if rupture occurs into the stomach or the superior pancreatico-duodenal artery if the cyst ruptures into the duodenum.

3 Rupture into the peritoneum causing ascites, or into the pleural cavity causing a pleural effusion.

The most serious of these complications is haemorrhage; over half the patients developing this complication die.

Question Should all pancreatic pseudocysts be operated upon immediately.

Answer No. Most observers agree that all cysts under 4 cm in diameter should be treated conservatively and all cysts following diagnosis should be left to mature for a period of between four and six weeks. If the patient is unable to eat intravenous nutrition should be continued throughout this period. A variable percentage of cysts will spontaneously resolve, figures of 30 per cent being quoted in the surgical literature.

Question What surgical options are available once a decision to operate has been made.

Answer First, assuming that the underlying cause of the attack is biliary tract disease the gall bladder should be removed and an operative cholangiogram performed in order to establish that the duct is free from debris or calculi.

Second, the cyst must be drained. If this is performed by external drainage prolonged drainage will ensue, but eventually, assuming no obstruction exists in the head of the pancreas spontaneous closure of the fistula occurs.

Alternatively, the cyst may be drained into the stomach, duodenum or jejunum. If drained into the jejunum a Roux loop must be constructed.

The two commonest methods of treatment are external drainage and cystogastrostomy.

Question What mortality rate can be expected.

Answer Figures between 6 and 20 per cent are quoted in the literature. The chief causes of death being uncontrolled infection and haemorrhage. The author has seen two patients in whom following cysto-gastrostomy severe bleeding led to death.

Question Can pseudocysts recur following surgical drainage.

Answer Yes, but rarely.

Comment This patient was explored through a midline incision. A cholecystectomy was performed followed by a cholangiogram which was negative. The pseudocyst appeared to be above the lesser curve of the stomach and in separating the inferior surface of the liver from the lesser curve a hole was made in the lesser sac through which the cyst contents drained. The vessels of the lesser curve of the stomach were then divided and a gastrotomy wound made on the lesser curvature. The edges of this incision were then sutured to the torn edge of the lesser omentum by two layers of continuous Dexon. Despite the fall in serum calcium in the early stages of his disease no visible fat necrosis was present within the abdomen.

Post-operatively severe pulmonary problems marred his recovery. These were treated with antibiotics appropriate to the sensitivity of the organisms found in his sputum.

On the 17th post-operative day parenteral nutrition was stopped. However, following recovery from his pulmonary complications he developed an intermittent fever with an associated leucocytosis. A series of ultrasound examinations were performed, a typical result being shown in Fig. 12.5.

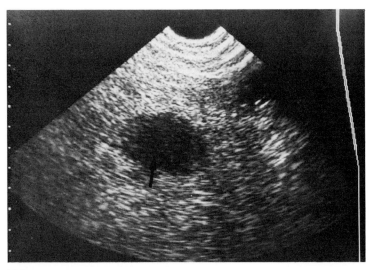

12.5

Question What does Fig. 12.5 show.
Answer An abscess cavity which was situated in the left flank.

Comment There was considerable debate as to whether this cavity should be aspirated or drained externally but serial examinations showed that a gradual reduction in the size of the cavity was occurring and it was finally decided to do nothing. A slow improvement occurred

120

and he was discharged from hospital on the 29th day following his laparotomy.

Seen three months later he was gaining weight and suffering no abdominal pain.

13

A Caucasian female, 50 years of age, was admitted complaining of severe right-sided upper abdominal pain associated with nausea and almost continuous vomiting of three days duration.

Her previous medical history was as follows:

1 30 years prior to admission she had suffered from acute appendicitis which had been treated surgically.

2 10 years prior to admission she had suffered from a prolonged period of abdominal pain. This had been thoroughly investigated and finally after a series of negative results a laparotomy had been performed. This had revealed no abnormality.

3 Seven years prior to admission an abdominal hysterectomy had been performed because of persistent menorrhagia.

4 Five years prior to admission she had complained of persistent diarrhoea. It was noted that the patient was nervous and depressed. No physical signs suggesting organic disease were found and no evidence of malabsorption was present. However, at the time of physical examination it was noted that she had some loss of sensation in both feet and legs together with loss of the ankle jerks and it finally emerged that she had been drinking heavily. A diagnosis of chronic alcoholism associated with diarrhoea and peripheral neuropathy was made. The patient and her relatives were warned of the dangers and she was treated for the neuropathy.

Examination on this admission Inspection revealed a thin almost emaciated female with three visible scars on her abdomen.

Abdominal examination	Palpation revealed tenderness in the right loin and rigidity across the whole of the upper abdomen.
Cardiovascular system	Negative. PR 80. BP 130/80.
Nervous system	Absent ankle jerks.

Comment The initial differential diagnosis appeared to be:

1 Subacute intestinal obstruction due to adhesions.

2 Right-sided renal colic.

3 Acute pancreatitis.

Question What are the chief features of polyneuritis due to alcoholism.

Answer Alcoholic neuropathy causes a polyneuropathy which usually begins distally and spreads proximally equally affecting both motor and sensory fibres. Paraesthesia and sensory loss of a stocking and glove type develop together with distal motor loss, the latter causing obvious wasting and weakness leading to foot drop in the lower limbs and impaired function of the hands in the upper limb.

Question What vitamin deficiencies occur in alcoholics.

Answer

1 Vitamin C.

2 Thiamine.

3 Folic acid.

Question What treatment is necessary.

Answer These vitamins should be replaced. Thiamine can be given as Becosyn Syrup (Roche UK) which also contains various other vitamins of the B group. Vitamin C can be given as a tablet (Roscorbic (Roche UK)) and folic acid as folic acid tablets (BP).

Comment The following investigations were ordered:

1 Full Blood Count: Hb, 15.3 g/dl, total nucleated cell count, predominantly polymorphonuclear leucocytes, $16.2 \times 10^9/l$.

3 Ultrasound of the gall bladder and pancreas: this revealed the presence of gall-stones.

4 Serum amylase: 3600 Somoygi units, all other biochemical tests revealed no abnormality.

These results appear to confirm the diagnosis of acute pancreatitis and the patient was treated by nasogastric suction and intravenous fluids. Within three days the patient was symptom free and she was discharged to await readmission in 12 weeks time for cholecystectomy. However, eight weeks after discharge she was readmitted complaining of right upper quadrant pain, vomiting and loss of weight of six weeks duration. The pain was also present in the back and was sufficiently severe to prevent sleep.

Physical examination revealed an emaciated woman. There was no evidence of jaundice. Abdominal examination revealed tenderness particularly in the right upper quadrant.

The biochemical tests previously performed were repeated and revealed that the serum amylase was still grossly elevated, being 2800 Somogyi units.

Question What does this suggest.

Answer Chronic pancreatitis with possible gastric outlet obstruction.

Question What is the present internationally accepted classification of pancreatitis.

Answer The Second International Symposium on the Concepts and Classification of Pancreatitis (1984) suggested that pancreatitis should be classified as acute or chronic, thus replacing the older classification suggested at the first Marseille conference in 1963 which was as follows: acute pancreatitis, relapsing acute pancreatitis, chronic relapsing pancreatitis and chronic pancreatitis.

Chronic pancreatitis as defined in 1984 at the Marseille conference is a disease characterized by recurrent or persisting abdominal pain, although recognizing that chronic pancreatitis may not necessarily be associated with pain. Pancreatic insufficiency producing steatorrhoea or diabetes may be present. The morphological changes characteristic of chronic pancreatitis are defined as:

Chronic pancreatitis with focal necrosis.

Chronic pancreatitis with segmental or diffuse fibrosis.

Chronic pancreatitis with or without calculi.

In chronic pancreatitis it was agreed that progressive or permanent loss of exocrine and endocrine pancreatic function may develop and that both the structural and functional changes may improve, if the obstruction is removed.

Comment Following admission the patient required narcotics for the relief of her intermittent epigastric and lower thoracic back pain. The serum amylase varied between 1520–3200 Somoygi units.

Question What tests of pancreatic exocrine functions have been described.
Answer Exocrine function may be measured by the following tests:

1 The secretin or secretin—cholecystokinin test. The disadvantages of this test are that it has not yet been standardized. There is, for example, no general agreement as to how the pancreas should be stimulated, how the secretions should be collected and what should be measured. Many investigators consider that to give secretin alone is sufficient rather than secretin together with cholecystokinin. The majority have found that the bicarbonate output is less variable than the enzyme output and that estimation of the latter is neither essential nor does it add to the diagnostic capability of the test.

In chronic pancreatitis a gross reduction in hourly volume of pancreatic secretion is found together with a reduction in the bicarbonate concentration.

2 Lundl test. This test is probably of greater value than the secretin test. The test meal administered provides a physiological stimulus for the endogenous release of pancreatic hormones.

The fasting patient is intubated and the position of the tube which must be present in the duodenum or upper jejunum is verified by radiological means. A test meal is then given, this should be around 300 ml in volume and contain five per cent fat, five per cent protein and 15 per cent carbohydrate. After the administration of the meal the duodenal contents are collected for two hours either by siphonage or mechanical suction in four half-hourly samples. Total recovery of duodenal juice is unnecessary because it is the concentration of enzymes, normally trypsin, which is measured.

Chronic pancreatic disease is associated with a marked fall in tryptic activity. The normal mean tryptic activity is between 27–80 μmol/ml/min whereas in chronic pancreatic disease this falls to between 0–27 μmol/ml/min.

As with the secretin test the Lundl test cannot help to differentiate chronic pancreatitis from carcinoma of the pancreas.

3 An indirect test of pancreatic function is the measurement of the faecal fat which is a measure of lipase excretion. This test is a timed faecal fat collection. It is performed by placing the patient on a standardized fat intake, usually 100 g daily and then saving the stools for a three day period.

The beginning and the end of the period should be marked either by the oral administration of charcoal or carmine red or alternatively a continuous marker such as chromium oxide or barium sulphate can be given. Thus when 1 g of the last compound is administered daily and the subsequent stool collection contains 3 g it can be safely assumed that a true three day collection has been made. If the amount of fat consumed is also known a ratio between excretion and intake can be calculated. The coefficient of fat absorption is

$$\frac{\text{intake} - \text{excretion}}{\text{intake}} \times 100$$

This should be greater than 93 per cent. Thus on a daily intake of 100 g of fat less than 7 g should be excreted daily.

The use of this test is limited by the simple fact that steatorrhoea only occurs when more than 95 per cent of the pancreatic tissue has been destroyed. Investigation has shown that only about 20 per cent of patients suffering from chronic pancreatitis have a diminished coefficient of fat absorption.

Question How can a minimal defect in fat absorption be enhanced.

Answer Since, in malabsorption, the total fat in the stools is proportional to the intake a minimal defect in fat absorption can usually be made more obvious by increasing the intake of fat.

Comment In this patient a normal coefficient of fat absorption was found on a dietary intake of 150 g daily.

Question What is the simplest test of pancreatic endocrine function.

Answer Measurement of the fasting blood sugar. In this patient the result was 9.5 mmol/l (N 3.4–5.0 mmol/l).

Question What does this suggest.

Answer That the β cells in the Islet of Langerhans are functioning imperfectly

Comment No palpable mass developed in the abdomen in this patient despite the raised amylase and a total nucleated cell count in excess of 20×10^9/l. Fifteen days following admission a further ultrasound examination of the pancreas was ordered. This showed the possible presence of a calculus in the head of the pancreas but no evidence of pseudocyst or pancreatic abscess.

Question What is the composition of pancreatic stones.

Answer The chief component of pancreatic calculi is calcium carbonate. This mineral is bound by a protein and a mixture of several polysaccharides. Under normal conditions pancreatic protein prevents the precipitation of the calcium carbonate with which pancreatic juice is normally supersaturated.

Question What investigation will localize the site of the pancreatic calcifications.

Answer Endoscopic retrograde cholangio-pancreatography introduced by the Japanese workers Ogoshi, Tobita and Hara in 1970.

Comment This was performed. The duodenum was found to be narrowed by oedema, the ampulla was located and successfully cannulated. Urografin 310 M was injected into the ductal system.

Question The results of this investigation are shown in Figs 13.1, 13.2 and 13.3. What do these radiographs show.

Answer The presence of a single large stone within the pancreatic duct together with proximal dilatation of the duct in the body of the gland.

Comment One month following admission despite commencing parenteral nutrition 14 days previously the patient was still complaining of severe pain. The serum amylase remained in excess of 2000 units and the leucocytosis persisted.

Question Is obstruction of the pancreatic duct an important cause of pancreatic pain.

Answer Apparently not necessarily so. An investigation performed by Bornman and his colleagues, reported in the *British Journal of Surgery* (1980), suggested that obstruction of the pancreatic duct by

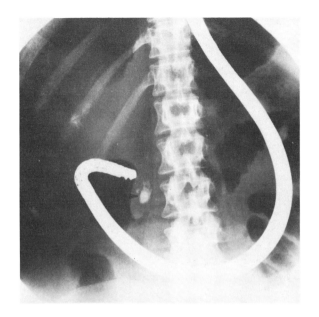

13.1

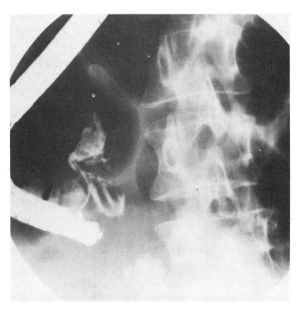

13.2

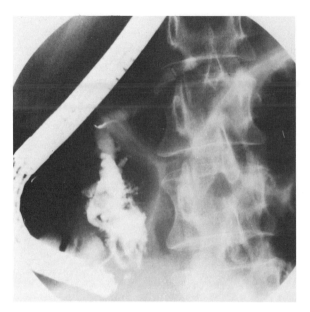

13.3

either a calculus or a stricture was not a significant cause of pancreatic pain. In a group of some 47 patients investigated at the Groote Schuur Gastroenterology unit they found that the incidence of pancreatic duct obstruction or stricture was of the same order in patients who were complaining of pain as those who were not.

Comment If the duct draining a gland is obstructed, two pathological consequences may follow. Either atrophy or infection proximal to the obstruction. Therefore, as a general principle, if possible, the obstruction should be relieved.

Question How can obstruction of the pancreatic duct be relieved.
Answer The idea of drainage of the pancreas as a cure for pancreatitis was first advanced by Link in 1911 who performed the operation of pancreatostomy, i.e. he produced an external pancreatic fistula. The difficulties of managing this fistula led to this operation being abandoned.

In 1956, Doubilet and Mulholland published a large series of cases of chronic pancreatitis in which they claimed many of the symptoms had been relieved by sphincterotomy. Since their results were never duplicated this operation also fell into disrepute.

128

In 1958, Peustow and Gillesby suggested and performed an extensive drainage procedure in the following manner:

1 The pancreas is mobilized after performing a splenectomy.
2 The tail is removed in order to identify the duct.
3 The pancreas is divided along its anterior face opening up the pancreatic duct medially.
4 A fillet of pancreatic tissue is removed to try and prevent reunion of the divided duct.
5 The tail and body of the pancreas is ensheathed by a jejunal loop.

In 1960, Partigan and Rochelle modified this last operation in order to avoid:

1 The performance of a splenectomy.
2 The extensive dissection necessary to mobilize the pancreas from the retroperitoneal tissues.

In their procedure the duct is laid open. The end of a Roux en Y loop of jejunum is bevelled by dividing it along its antimesenteric border after which it is stitched to the pancreas in such a manner that it covers the opened pancreatic duct like a roof.

Comment Both the Puestow/Gillesby and the Partington/Rochelle modification appear to produce similar results, i.e. relief of pain occurs in approximately 70 per cent of patients. However, it undoubtedly appears that the best results are achieved in alcoholic pancreatitis if, in addition to a drainage procedure, the patient abstains from alcohol.

Question Does surgery retard the development of exocrine and endocrine deficiencies.
Answer Examination of the literature suggests that the natural history of the disease remains unchanged after drainage procedures. Certainly many investigators have found no improvement in fat and nitrogen absorption following surgery. The improved nutrition which follows surgery is probably due to the relief of pain rather than improvement in pancreatic function.
Question What is known about the long term patency of the anastomoses described.
Answer In one study performed by Potts *et al.* and reported in the *American Journal of Surgery* (1981) it was found by post-operative ERCP that following caudal pancreatico-jejunostomy occlusion of the anastomosis occurred but that this was not followed by recurrent pain.

Comment In this patient laparotomy was performed 26 days after her second admission. The chief operative findings were:

1 Gross fat necrosis especially in the omentum.
2 A thin walled gall bladder containing a few pigment stones.
3 A normal common bile duct containing no stones.
4 A grossly thickened pancreas.

Procedure The tail and body of the pancreas were dissected free. The tail of the pancreas was then removed and the pancreatic duct was traced medially towards the head. The duct was grossly dilated and a spiculated calcium carbonate stone lay within the duct 2 cm distal to the ampulla. There was a marked reaction around the stone which was removed following which a pancreatico-jejunostomy was performed.

The patient required intensive care for pulmonary difficulties immediately following surgery with intubation and positive pressure ventilation being necessary until the third post-operative day. Gradual recovery then occurred, the patient being discharged on the sixteenth post-operative day.

Question What final diagnosis would you suggest.

Answer Pancreatitis due to alcoholism complicated by the formation of a pancreatic calculus.

14

A 22-year-old Caucasian male was admitted complaining of increasing abdominal pain for five days. The pain was central at its onset and described by the patient as sharp. Two days after its commencement the pain moved to the right iliac fossa becoming more severe and at the same time he developed right shoulder tip pain which, although present all the time, was made worse by coughing. Throughout this illness he had been anorexic. The bowels were opened daily and he had no dysuria.

Social habits He drinks 10 pints of beer a week and smokes 20 cigarettes a day.

Past medical history Seven years prior to the present admission he had suffered attacks of severe abdominal pain for a period of some weeks which had been associated with a sore throat and fever.

Physical examination

Respiratory system	Normal. Respiratory rate 20/min.
Alimentary tract	The tongue was furred. Abdominal palpation revealed tenderness extending from the level of the right costal margin to the right iliac fossa.
Rectal examination	Tenderness present in the Pouch of Douglas.
Cardiovascular system	PR 80/min, BP 120/70.
Temperature	38.8°C.

Question What is the presumptive diagnosis.

Answer Acute appendicitis. However, the complaint of *right* shoulder tip pain in a patient suffering from acute appendicitis is difficult to explain in the absence of signs of general peritonitis. After five days, in the majority of patients suffering from acute appendicitis, either localization of the inflammatory process has occurred or rupture has led to a general diffuse peritonitis.

Question What physical signs have been described which support a diagnosis of acute appendicitis.

Answer Several signs have been described but no physical sign positively confirms the diagnosis; all merely indicate that an acute inflammatory lesion is present in the right iliac fossa or pelvis.

    1   Cope's sign. Flexion and internal rotation of the right hip. If the

inflamed appendix is in close relation to the obturator internus this movement will cause pain.

2 Psoas sign. Extension of the right hip may cause pain when the diseased organ lies in close relationship to this muscle.

3 Cutaneous hyperaesthesia. If the parietal peritoneum also becomes involved in the inflammatory process hyperaesthesia develops in the skin superficial to the affected area. In appendicitis the area of hyperaesthesia is usually limited to Sherren's triangle. In this patient, in view of the physical signs described one might reasonably have expected to find cutaneous hyperaesthesia over the whole of the right side of the abdomen and possibly over the tip of the right shoulder.

Question What special investigations may be helpful in confirming the presumptive diagnosis of acute appendicitis.

Answer

1 Plain X-ray of the abdomen. In approximately 50 per cent of patients suffering from acute appendicitis some abnormality will be seen in a plain abdominal X-ray film. The two most common signs are:

(a) distension of distal loops of ileum present in the right iliac fossa.

(b) an increase in the density of the soft tissue of the wall and base of the caecum.

2 Haematological examination. Since all laboratories in the Western World are using a Coulter counter a measurement of all the cellular constitutents of the blood is obtained.

The white blood count can be expected to be raised in about one-half of all patients suffering from acute appendicitis but it is generally conceded that should the clinical findings be at variance with the count the former should take precedence in the clinician's thinking. In this patient, because the physical signs indicated an extensive inflammatory process one would be surprised if it were not raised.

The result was as follows:

RBC – 4.39×10^{12}/l.

Hb – 12.4 g/dl.

Total nucleated cell count – l 81.3×10^9/l.

Platelet count – 31×10^9/l.

Question Can you comment on this result.

Answer This result is so grossly abnormal that it suggests a previously unrecognized granulocytic leukaemia is present in addition to the normal response to an acute inflammatory condition. However, the pronounced reactive neutrophilia sometimes associated with infection can occasionally cause a blood picture closely resembling that of chronic myeloid leukaemia.

Comment At this stage, however, the obvious infective lesion takes precedence over all other problems.

Question What incision would you make.

Answer The correct incision is undoubtedly a right paramedian since the presence of tenderness over the whole of the right side of the abdomen indicates that the inflammatory lesion has spread and in addition the complaint of right shoulder tip pain suggests that a right suprahepatic abscess may be developing.

Question What condition other than a developing right suprahepatic abscess might produce shoulder tip pain in a patient suffering from acute appendicitis.

Answer Multiple liver abscesses following a portal pyaemia or an ascending pylephlebitis.

Question What are the common causes of liver abscess other than acute appendicitis.

Answer
1 Ascending cholangitis due to infection in the biliary tree.
2 Diverticulitis.
3 In endemic areas, *Entamoeba histolytica*.

Comment The operative findings were as follows:
1 No free fluid in the abdomen.
2 An inflamed pelvic appendix which was sent for histology, this confirmed the presence of acute appendicitis.
3 Multiple nodules in the liver.

Question What procedures would you perform.
Answer
1 Appendicectomy.
2 Incise or excise one or more of the liver nodules. In attempting the latter the nodule ruptured, pus exuded from the surface of the liver. This was then sent for culture.

The corrected surgical diagnosis is, therefore, acute appendicitis associated with portal pyaemia. The operative findings explain the physical signs. The shoulder tip pain is due to irritation of the parietal peritoneum on the under surface of the diaphragm by abscesses present on the upper surface of the right lobe of the liver.

Question Is portal pyaemia common.

Answer No. The incidence of this complication of acute appendicitis has fallen due to two factors:
1 The earlier diagnosis of the disease and, therefore, earlier treatment.

133

2 The introduction of antibiotics.

However, septicaemia, pyaemia, and opportunistic infections remain relatively common in patients with lowered resistance to bacterial infection, for example in patients suffering from agranulocytosis, immunodeficient states and therapeutic immunosuppression.

Question Is the risk of infection greater in chronic granulocytic leukaemia and if the answer is yes, what are the commonest pathogens found.

Answer Yes. The commonest organisms causing severe infection in chronic granulocytic leukaemia are:

1 *Staphylococcus aureus.*
2 *Escherichia coli.*
3 *Pseudomonas aeruginosa.*

Question Why is infection particularly dangerous in chronic granulocytic leukaemia.

Answer Because:

1 The neutrophils are less effective than in a normal individual. This can be proven by a variety of tests, particularly by their inability to ingest *Candida albicans.*

2 The granulocytes have a decreased adhesiveness making them unable to concentrate at foci of infection.

Question Assuming as yet, without actual proof, that this patient is suffering from portal pyaemia together with chronic granulocytic leukaemia what antibiotics should be administered.

Answer

1 Gentamicin. 80 mg, eight hourly intravenously.
2 Metranidazole. 500 mg, eight hourly intravenously.
3 Ampicillin. 250 mg, six hourly intramuscularly.

Question What precautions should be taken when administering the aminoglycoside.

Answer The blood levels should be checked daily to confirm that the peak (one hour) levels do not exceed 10 mcg/ml and that the trough levels, one hour prior to the injection, do not exceed 2 mcg/ml.

If levels in excess of 10 mcg/ml are achieved, as might occur in the severely ill patient or in patients suffering from renal failure, vestibular toxicity may occur.

Question What other toxic manifestations of gentamicin have been reported.

Answer

1 Neuromuscular blockage.
2 Respiratory paralysis in patients receiving curare-like drugs during anaesthesia.

Question Why is metranidazole being administered.

Answer Because the primary source of the infection in this patient is from the gut it is, therefore, reasonable to presume that *Bacteriodes fragilis* and *fuseformis* will be present in the liver abscesses.

Question In view of the operative findings what biochemical abnormalities might be present and what, if any, would be their predictive value.

Answer

1 The most important are tests designed to indicate the presence of parenchymal liver damage. These are the estimation of the glutamic oxaloacetic transaminase and glutamic pyruvic transaminase, both enzymes found in the liver. A rise in these enzymes, found as anticipated in this case, indicates the presence of parenchymal liver damage. A continuing rise would indicate increasing hepatic destruction and in this patient failure, therefore, to control infection. In this patient the GOT (AST) whilst raised for approximately one week fell to normal during the second.

2 Serum bilirubin. In this case the serum bilirubin remained within normal limits, any rise would indicate increasing damage to the liver.

Question What non-invasive technique allows the anatomical changes in the liver to be followed.

Answer Abdominal ultrasound. One day after admission, ultrasonography demonstrated ill-defined areas of abnormal liver texture consistent with early abscess formation. Four days later multiple small echo poor focal areas with surrounding bright areas were present, a finding consistent with multiple small abscesses. The changes as anticipated were chiefly in the right lobe of the liver. Fifteen days later although the liver remained enlarged these changes had resolved.

Question How does one confirm the diagnosis of chronic granulocytic leukaemia.

Answer

1 Following the control of the infection the white count would remain high.

2 Repeated granulocyte counts should demonstrate the presence of metamyelocytes.

3 The neutrophil alkaline phosphatase score should be high.

4 Chromosomal analysis of the granulocytes should show the presence of the Philadelphia chromosome.

Question What is the Philadelphia chromosome.

Answer This is a consistent structural chromosomal aberration consisting of the small G chromosomal deletion in the white and red blood cell precursors in the marrow.

Comment In this patient the Philadelphia chromosome was present confirming the diagnosis of chronic granulocytic leukaemia.

Question How is chronic granulocytic leukaemia normally treated.

Answer By the administration of busulphan, 4 mg daily up to a maximum yearly dose of between 400–700 mg. Because the destruction of white blood cells gives rise to raised blood uric acid levels gout may occur and to avoid this allopurinol 100 mg three times a day by mouth should be administered.

Question What are the causes of death in chronic granulocytic leukaemia.

Answer

1 Intracranial haemorrhage, the high leucocyte count and low platelet count predispose to bleeding.

2 Overwhelming gram −ve septicaemia, particularly in hospitalized patients.

In this patient recovery occurred and the patient was discharged 20 days following admission and has remained well on chemotherapy for one year.

15

A Caucasian male, aged 17, was admitted complaining of increasingly severe abdominal pain of six months duration together with the loss of 9 kilograms in weight. The pain, colicky in nature, was situated in the periumbilical region. It was precipitated by taking food but not fluids and was associated with borborgymi and a feeling of distension. Normally lasting for several minutes, on occasion it would take about one hour before relief occurred. His appetite had virtually disappeared. His bowels were loose, with 3–4 motions a day, yellow in colour, for several weeks prior to admission.

Previous medical history None.

Abdominal examination Inspection: no abnormality. Palpation: vague tenderness in the right iliac fossa. Auscultation: negative at the time of examination but re-examined after food the bowel sounds were exaggerated and obstructive in type. PR: negative.

All other systems negative.

Question What does the history suggest.

Answer Chronic small bowel obstruction.

Question What is the commonest cause of progressive small bowel obstruction in a young person.

Answer Crohn's disease.

Question When did Crohn first describe the disease known by his name.

Answer In 1932. He then described the condition as affecting the terminal ileum only, thus the original descriptive term applied to the disease, 'regional ileitis'. Somewhat later it was recognized that the disease could affect the jejunum, hence the term regional enteritis. Now it is appreciated that any part of the gastrointestinal tract from the mouth to the anus can be affected, hence the use of the term Crohn's disease, a term which embraces not only the gastrointestinal manifestations of the disease but also the peripheral phenomena.

Question What is known about the aetiology of Crohn's disease.

Answer The aetiology of Crohn's disease remains unknown. Genetic predisposition is important, a high concordance rate has been observed in monozygotic as opposed to dizygotic twins. In the United States it is commoner in Caucasians than Blacks and commoner in Jews than non-Jews. In fact Crohn originally believed he was describing a disease entity specifically affecting Jews.

The granulomatous lesions and the lymphocytic infiltration seen in Crohn's disease suggests an immune mechanism and in keeping with this hypothesis many immunological changes have been described. For example, increased K-cell activity is present in patients suffering from Crohn's disease who have not been treated by immunosuppressive drugs.

Question How would you define diarrhoea.

Answer An increase in the frequency of, or a decrease in the consistency of the stool or both.

Question What are the chief physiological causes of diarrhoea.

Answer Diarrhoea may result from:

1 Osmotic disturbance.
2 Secretory disturbance.
3 Damage to the intestinal mucosa.
4 Deranged intestinal motility.

Question Which of these causes the diarrhoea associated with Crohn's disease.

Answer All may be involved:

1 If sufficient destruction of the intestinal mucosa has occurred or if blind loops have developed a secondary lactase deficiency results in osmotic diarrhoea.
2 An excess of dehydroxy bile acids reaching the colon induces a secretory disturbance.
3 Malabsorption of fat may follow damage to the intestinal mucosa.
4 Intestinal motility is disturbed by:
a Ulceration and inflammation of the intestinal mucosa.
b Abnormal flora in blind loops.
c The development of internal fistula.
d Strictures.

Question What investigations would you require to confirm the diagnosis of Crohn's disease.

Answer The principle investigation required is a small bowel enema.

Question What are the most reliable radiological signs of Crohn's disease.

Answer

1 Ulceration and irregularity of the mucosa.
2 Clefts in the wall of the bowel.
3 Contraction.
4 Rigidity.
5 Cobblestone appearance.

Comment The small bowel meal in this patient is shown in Figs 15.1 and 15.2. This clearly shows an extensive cobblestone appearance of the terminal ileum together with clefts in the wall of the bowel. Rigidity and contraction can only be appreciated by the radiologist at the time of the examination.

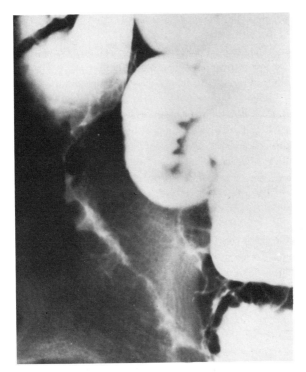

15.1

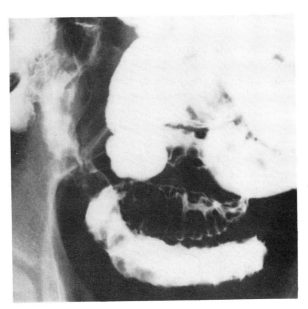

15.2

139

Question What other investigations would be of value.

Answer

    1 Erythrocyte sedimentation rate. This is one of the most satisfactory ways of determining the activity of the disease.

    2 Full blood count. An iron deficiency anaemia is not uncommon in Crohn's disease because of mucosal bleeding. Less commonly but particularly when the disease affects the terminal ileum both a folic acid and Vitamin B_{12} deficiency might occur due to malabsorption causing a macrocytic anaemia.

    3 Estimation of the faecal fat. Fat absorption may be found defective in severe and extensive disease of the terminal ileum.

Question What are the chief macroscopic features of intestinal Crohn's disease.

Answer

    1 'Hose-pipe' strictures of the small bowel or colon due to the abnormal thickness of the gut wall. The strictures may be short or long, single or multiple.

    2 Ulceration of the mucosa. The earliest lesion is an apthous ulcer, whereas in the later stages of the disease the ulcers become deep fissures passing through all layers of the bowel wall.

    3 A 'cobble-stone' appearance of the mucosa caused by the inter-communicating fissures surrounding islands of mucous membrane raised up by underlying inflammation and oedema.

    4 Enlargement of adjacent lymph nodes.

Question What are the chief histological features of Crohn's disease.

Answer

    1 A sarcoid or tuberculoid reaction in the affected tissues and regional lymph nodes. Each granuloma is composed of epithelioid cells within which giant cells of the Langhan's type are found. Precisely similar lesions are found in the regional lymph nodes.

    2 Fissuring, consisting of knife-like clefts which extend downwards to involve the entire thickness of the wall of the bowel. Each is lined by granulation tissue and sometimes by epithelioid cells together with giant cells of both the Langhan's and foreign body type.

    3 Transmural inflammation of the whole thickness of the bowel wall within which may be found focal collections of lymphocytes.

Question Is the disease limited to solitary or multiple areas of involvement of the gastrointestinal tract.

Answer No. Histological and functional tests indicate that Crohn's disease affects the entire gastrointestinal tract. Biopsy morphometry of the proximal jejunum, in patients suffering from disease of the distal ileum, shows that there is a reduction, in the apparently healthy gut, of the surface area. In addition enzyme studies indicate a significant reduction in disaccharidase in the brush border throughout the bowel. It has also been shown by Truelove and his co-workers that the mucosa of the rectum taken from patients suffering from ileal disease has a significantly increased plasma cell density in the lamina propria, in the volume of the lamina propria and in glucosamine-synthetase activity.

Question What lesions outside the gastrointestinal tract occur in Crohn's disease.

Answer Chiefly skin lesions in which granulomata can be identified. Other lesions not associated with granulomata include:

1 Pyoderma gangrenosum.
2 Erythema nodosum and multiforme.
3 Eczema.
4 The ulceration of Behçet's syndrome.

Other than skin lesions, patients suffering from Crohn's disease suffer a higher than normal chance of developing ankylosing spondylitis and polyarthritis.

Question What are the chief surgical complications of Crohn's disease.

Answer

1 Subacute intestinal obstruction due to the development of strictures.
2 Internal fistula formation due to transmural inflammation and serosal reaction.
3 External fistula formation, this type of fistula may occur spontaneously but much more frequently follows resection of diseased areas of gut.
4 Fistula *in ano,* tags, fissures and abscesses.

Question What is the chief clinical characteristic of the anal lesions associated with Crohn's disease.

Answer Despite the appearance of great severity they seldom cause severe symptoms.

Question What is the frequency of anal lesions.

Answer Anal lesions occur in a very high proportion of patients suffering from Crohn's disease, in some recorded series as high as 80 per cent and in many patients the development of an anal lesion precedes the onset of intestinal symptoms by some years.

Question What factor appears to govern the frequency of anal lesions.

Answer The site of the disease. When the disease primarily involves the small bowel the percentage of patients suffering from anal disease varies according to the series examined between 11 and 76 per cent whereas in colonic disease, the percentage varies between 50 and 93 per cent and when the rectum is involved the incidence of anal lesions rises to 100 per cent.

Question Will the anal lesion heal when treated in the appropriate manner by surgery.

Answer Yes, unless the colon is involved.

Question What oro-facial lesions can occur in Crohn's disease.

Answer

1 Angular cheilitis.
2 Mucosal tags.
3 Cobblestoning of the oral mucosa.
4 Hyperplastic gingival lesions.
5 Oral ulcers.

Question Can the course of Crohn's disease be systematically plotted.

Answer Yes, by the use of indices such as the Crohn's disease Activity Index.

Question Define the parameters used in the CDAI.

Answer The development of the index depends on eight predictor variables. An index of 150 or less indicates quiescent disease, between 160–440 active disease and above 450 severe disease.

The variables used are as follows:

	Factor Subtotal
1 No. of liquid or very soft stools over a seven day period	$\times 2 =$
2 Abdominal pain over seven days judged to be: 0–1, mild; 2, moderate; 3, severe	$\times 5 =$
3 General well-being over seven days: 0, good; 1, slightly under par; 2, poor; 3, very poor; 4, terrible.	$\times 7 =$
4 Add listed categories suffered by the patient: (a) Arthritis/arthralgia (b) Iritis/uveitis. (c) Erythema nodosum/pyoderma Apthous stomatitis (d) Anal fissure/fistula/abscess. (e) Other fistula. (f) Fever over 38°C	$\times 20 =$
5 Taking antidiarrhoeal. 0 = No 1 = Yes	$\times 30 =$
6 Abdominal mass. 0 = No 2 = questionable 5 = definite	$\times 10 =$
7 Haemacrit. Males 47 – Subtotal Females 42 – add or subtract	$\times 6 =$
8 Body weight. Percentage below standard weight	$\times 1 =$

Comment In this patient the CDAI was 320, indicating moderate to severe disease.

Since this index is a somewhat cumbersome method of assessment other less complicated methods have been suggested. For example, a clinical assessment based on such parameters as well-being, the presence or absence of pain, diarrhoea and complications combined with such simple non-specific laboratory indicators, the most important of which are the degree of elevation of the ESR and C-reactive protein.

Question What forms of medical treatment have been used in Crohn's disease.

Answer A variety of drugs and regimes have been used. These include prednisolone, Salazopyrine, azathioprine, 6-Mercaptopurine, the use of an elemental diet and total parenteral nutrition and a variety of antibiotics including framycetin and colistin.

Comment In the National Co-operative Crohn's Disease Study performed in America it was found that both prednisolone and Salazopyrine were more effective in controlling active disease than was a placebo. Salazopyrine appeared to be the drug of choice in the previously untreated patient and was less toxic than either prednisolone or azathioprine. When prednisolone and Salazopyrine were used together in active disease less improvement was recorded than with the use of prednisolone alone. However, neither prednisolone or Salazopyrine appeared to be of value in quiescent disease or following resection in preventing a recurrence. However, in contradistinction to some workers in this field it was found that azathioprine 2 mg/kg per day was of value in preventing a relapse following a remission induced by prednisolone.

Cooke found no long term benefit from the use of corticotrophin or corticosteroids and found that the risk of requiring an operation each year for patients treated with steroids was twice that of untreated patients.

Question What dose of prednisolone may be required.
Answer Up to 5 mg/kg per day.
Question What dose of Salazopyrine would you use.
Answer 1–2 g orally four times a day.
Question What are the chief indications for surgical treatment in Crohn's disease.
Answer
1 Obstruction.
2 Internal or external fistulae.
3 Chronic anaemia.

4 Abscess formation.

5 Rarely acute dilatation of the colon.

Question What would you do with this patient who was rapidly losing weight and suffering increasing pain.

Answer An ileal resection.

Comment The abdomen was explored through a right lower paramedian incision. The chief findings were as follows:

1 A 40 cm loop of ileum stretching proximally from the ileocaecal junction exhibited a typical 'hose pipe' appearance.

2 Proximal to this was a further 40 cm of bowel which was slightly dilated, the serosa was hyperaemic and small 'tubercles' were present beneath it.

Question What is the nature of the subserosal 'tubercles'.

Answer They are the sarcoid-like granulomata of Crohn's disease.

Question What operative choices are available.

Answer

1 Resect the strictured area together with the area of minimal involvement, a total resection of approximately 90–100 cm.

2 Resect the stricture leaving the bowel in which 'tubercles' are present.

3 Bypass the diseased bowel by performing an ileotransverse colostomy.

Question Is bypass surgery for Crohn's disease a viable method of treatment.

Answer No. The majority of large series report a significantly higher rate of recurrence of the disease following simple bypass procedures.

Comment In this patient the distal 60 cm of ileum together with the caecum and proximal 10 cm of the colon were resected and an end to end ileo-colic anastomosis performed. At the point of ileal transection the 'tubercles' were spare.

Question What are the reported rates of recurrence following resection for Crohn's disease.

Answer These vary according to the series examined but fairly typical findings are as follows: recurrent symptoms associated with radiological changes will develop in approximately one-third of all patients within five years and this will have increased to 50 per cent within 10 years. The severity of the recurrence is such that approximately 15 per cent of patients require a further resection within five years and 25 per cent within 10 years.

Question Does the age of the patient influence the incidence of recurrence.

Answer Yes. In several series it has been shown that the younger the patient at the time of the first operation the greater the incidence of recurrence.

Question Does microscopic evidence of disease at the point of resection influence the incidence of recurrence.

Answer Apparently not.

Comment The histological changes found in the resected specimen were typical of Crohn's disease. The caecum and colon were not involved and in the more proximal ileum some focal ulceration, scattered submucosal and subserosal granulomata were present. The patient made an uninterrupted recovery and was discharged on the twelfth post-operative day. However, when seen as an out-patient some six weeks later he was complaining of severe diarrhoea, his bowels being open 6–7 times a day.

Question What investigation is required.

Answer The patient's faecal fat should be estimated.

Question Why.

Answer Because there are two possible causes for the diarrhoea:

1 That it is due to the malabsorption of fat.

2 That it is due to failure of absorption of bile salts resulting in an increased concentration in the colon. This precipitates a watery diarrhoea.

Question What difference does this make to treatment.

Answer Diarrhoea due to the malabsorption of fat may be improved by a low fat diet whereas cholestyramine is required to overcome the effects of excessive quantities of bile salts reaching the colon.

Question What is the action of cholestyramine.

Answer Cholestyramine exchanges chloride ions for the anions of bile salts, which it binds into an insoluble complex. This is excreted in the faeces so preventing the normal reabsorption of bile salts. The dose is 4 g tds or qds falling to 1–2 g qds when relief has been achieved.

Comment In this patient fat absorption was within normal limits on a diet containing 150 g of fat daily and the patient was therefore given cholestyramine. Within three months he had regained the weight lost since the beginning of his illness.

Question Should this patient be followed up and if the answer is 'Yes', why.

Answer Yes, because he may:

1 Develop a recurrence.

2 Develop a macrocytic anaemia.

3 Develop other complications of Crohn's disease such as an entero-cutaneous fistula or a fistula *in ano.*

Comment The following is a history of a rather anxious introspective man who was first seen 14 years ago.

1972: aged 26, he was referred to the out-patient clinic complaining of four weeks of colicky central abdominal pain associated with anorexia and intermittent bilious vomiting. Twelve hours prior to admission the pain had localized in the right iliac fossa. Examination revealed that he was rigid and tender over the whole abdomen.

Laparotomy revealed the peritoneal cavity to be filled with turbid fluid. The appendix and caecum were normal but the terminal ileum was grossly thickened. A diagnosis of Crohn's disease was made, the appendix was removed and the abdomen closed without drainage.

A barium meal and follow through following recovery revealed a segment of Crohn's disease in the distal ileum. Three months later he developed a fistula *in ano* but was not complaining of abdominal pain.

1973: one year after the initial episode he returned with further abdominal pain and examination revealed a mass in the right iliac fossa. A barium enema revealed a fistula between the rectum and small bowel but despite this his symptoms rapidly settled following treatment with cortisone and bed rest.

1974: he was admitted complaining of severe pain in the back, right buttock and thigh, made worse on movement. In addition he complained of anorexia, insomnia and intermittent abdominal distension, and severe diarrhoea, all of approximately three and a half weeks duration. Examination revealed a temperature of 39°C, an abdominal mass in the right iliac fossa and on rectal examination a large 'boggy' mass posterior to the rectum. In the first operation, the retrorectal space was explored, large amounts of pus being released. This relieved his back pain but not the pain in the thigh. During the second operation the abdomen was explored and the terminal ileum was found matted together and adherent to the caecum. Within this mass was an abscess penetrating the psoas sheath. A further mass of small bowel was found adherent to the sigmoid although no obvious fistula was present. However, on separating the mass involving the terminal ileum several enteric fistula were found together with one loop fistulating into the rectum. A limited right hemicolectomy was performed together with a left iliac colostomy. The distal sigmoid was brought to the surface as a mucous fistula.

1975: both radiological and histological evidence of rectal disease was found thus precluding further surgery.

1976: an area of pyoderma gangrenosum developed which healed over a period of six months. He then remained well for three years.

1979: he was admitted complaining of colicky lower abdominal pain. An enema performed through the colostomy indicated a normal colon but the possibility of a mass compressing the terminal ileum. The small bowel enema showed severe recurrence of Crohn's disease with stenosis at the ileocolic junction and several intestinal fistulae.

He was treated with large doses of prednisolone and azathioprine. Two months later a further small bowel enema was carried out. Although once again it demonstrated typical areas of Crohn's disease, the obstructive element had greatly improved.

He was weaned from steroids but continued on azathioprine for one year.

1986: he was seen in outpatients with no abdominal complaints. His weight was normal.

This case illustrates the unpredictable course followed by this disease.

16

An obese 62-year-old married woman was admitted complaining of severe lower abdominal pain for 36 hours, at first across the whole of the lower abdomen but localizing to the left side of the abdomen from the rib cage downwards in the 12 hours prior to admission. The pain was described as severe and continuous. She had vomited repeatedly since the onset of the pain. From the onset she had had a constant desire to defaecate and had passed mucus and clots of fresh blood almost continuously for 24 hours prior to her admission.

Previous medical history Seven years prior to this admission she had suffered a similar but less severe attack which had undergone spontaneous remission. However, a barium enema and sigmoidoscopy had been performed, the former demonstrating scattered diverticuli in the sigmoid colon and the latter no abnormality.

Physical examination Inspection revealed a middle-aged woman who was obviously distressed and dehydrated.

Abdominal examination Palpation revealed generalized abdominal tenderness, much more marked in the left iliac fossa than elsewhere. Rebound tenderness and cutaneous hyperaesthesia were evident in the left iliac fossa.

Rectal examination Both mucus and blood were present on the finger.

Cardiovascular system BP 110/60. PR 90/minute. Heart not enlarged. Temperature 38.2°C.

Question What initial steps would you take.

Answer Correct the dehydration by intravenous therapy. Clinical dehydration is normally associated with a loss of 4 litres of fluid and 400 mmol of Na. Therefore, make every effort to correct this deficit but monitor the urine output and in an older patient take care that fluid overloading does not occur.

Question What is the differential diagnosis.

Answer
1 Diverticulitis, a diagnosis supported by the previous X-ray findings.
2 Inflammatory bowel disease.
3 Infectious colitis.
4 Ischaemic colitis.
5 Carcinoma of the colon.

Question Which of these diagnoses is the most probable.

Answer In view of the acute onset of the disease, infectious colitis or ischaemic colitis.

Question Since diverticuli has been previously demonstrated why should the diagnosis of diverticulitis be discarded.

Answer Mucosal bleeding, in patients suffering from diverticular disease, is commonly massive frequently producing 'clinical' shock or anaemia. It is rarely associated with any other symptoms.

Question What are the causes of infectious diarrhoea.

Answer Infectious diarrhoea is most commonly due to drinking contaminated water or eating contaminated food. In countries where this condition is common it may be avoided by refusing ice, salads and fruit. The common causes are:

1 The enterotoxigenic *Escherichia coli*.
2 Shigellosis, bacillary dysentery.
3 Giardia lamblia.

Less commonly:

1 *Salmonella typhi* and *paratyphi*.
2 Enteroviruses.
3 *Entamoeba histolytica*.
4 *Vibrio cholerae*.

Question What are the chief clinical features of infectious diarrhoea.

Answer

1 It is seldom restricted to an isolated case.
2 It is associated with the abrupt onset of severe vomiting and diarrhoea.
3 The faeces are watery in nature.

Question Which infections may cause blood and mucus in the stools.

Answer

1 *Shigella flexneri* and *dysenteriae* due to extensive ulceration of the colon.
2 Acute intestinal amoebiasis.

Question Which intestinal infections may result in perforation of the bowel:

Answer

1 *Shigella flexneri* and *dysenteriae* may rarely cause perforation of the colon.
2 *Salmonella typhi* may cause perforation of the small intestine.
3 Rarely acute amoebiasis.

Question What investigations would you order.

Answer

1 Electrolyte values.
2 Stool culture.
3 Plain X-ray of the abdomen.
4 Full blood count.

Comment The following results were obtained:

1 Electrolyte values: slight elevation of urea.
2 Stool culture: negative.
3 Plain X-ray: some gas in the right colon with a few fluid levels. No free gas under the diaphragm.
4 Full blood count: total nucleated cell count $14.1 \times 10^9/l$; RBC $4.86 \times 10^{12}/l$; Hb 13.4 g/dl.

Question How would you interpret these results.

Answer The leucocytosis establishes the presence of an intra-abdominal inflammatory lesion, the fluid levels in the right colon implying that there is an obstructive lesion present in the left colon.

Question Can the differential diagnosis be refined.

Answer Yes.

1 Infectious diarrhoea as an isolated event is rare in the UK although it is by no means uncommon in institutions.
2 Inflammatory bowel disease, i.e. Crohn's colitis and ulcerative colitis is only rarely associated with the acute presentation seen in this patient. She is in either case somewhat old to suffer from a first attack of either disease.

The differential diagnosis, therefore, is between:

(a) Diverticulitis.
(b) Carcinoma of the descending colon complicated by perforation and a developing pericolic abscess.
(c) Ischaemic colitis.

Comment A decision was made to treat the patient conservatively but after 48 hours there were no signs of improvement. The left side of the abdomen was now rigid and the rebound tenderness more marked. Laparotomy was, therefore, advised and performed. The chief findings were as follows:

1 A small amount of free fluid.
2 From the mid-transverse colon to the junction of the descending, with the sigmoid, the large bowel was grossly thickened and congested. Subserosal haemorrhages were present throughout the whole length of the affected gut and in three areas gangrenous changes were present.

Question What do these changes suggest.

Answer Ischaemic colitis. Ulcerative colitis normally commences in the rectum and spreads proximally without interruption. Although toxic dilatation may be associated with spontaneous perforation in this condition the entire colon is usually involved and whilst subserosal

150

haemorrhages may be present and the wall of the gut congested it is never thickened. One would anticipate finding a grossly distended bowel, the wall of which is thin with a tendency to tear when handled, like wet blotting paper.

Question What aetiological factors have been identified.

Answer

1 Arterial or venous thrombosis.

2 Embolism.

3 Various conditions in which small vessel disease occurs, e.g. polyarteritis nodosa and lupus erythematosus.

4 Non-occlusive vascular disease, e.g.

   (a) Hypovolaemic or septic shock.

   (b) Cardiac failure.

Question Do these aetiological factors account for the largest proportion of cases.

Answer No, the greater proportion of cases of ischaemic colitis are idiopathic, occurring spontaneously and with no apparent precipitating cause.

Question Does a plain X-ray of the abdomen ever demonstrate specific changes in this disease.

Answer Yes. A plain film would be diagnostic if it showed a segmental zone of the colon affected in which the bowel wall and the haustra were thickened together with proximal dilatation.

When infarction of the bowel has occurred bacterial invasion, by destroying the mucosal integrity, causes linear pneumatosis and possibly gas in the portal vein or when perforation of the colon has occurred, free air in the abdominal cavity.

Question What is the clinical spectrum presented by ischaemic colitis.

Answer The clinical spectrum varies between a trivial episode of abdominal pain and diarrhoea to the patient who rapidly develops 'shock' and a rigid abdomen due to gangrenous infarction of the bowel.

Question What factors determine where she or he falls in the clinical spectrum.

Answer

1 The duration of ischaemia.

2 The efficiency of the collateral circulation.

3 The extent of bacterial invasion.

Question Is the rectum ever involved in this disease.

Answer Never in the naturally occurring disease because of the abundant collateral circulation but an ischaemic rectal lesion very occasionally follows ligation of the inferior mesenteric artery during the course of reconstructive aorto-iliac surgery.

151

Question Is a barium enema ever justified in this disease.

Answer Yes, in milder forms of the disease, thus it was contra-indicated in this patient because the physical signs were those associated with a developing peritonitis.

Question What are the classical radiological signs associated with ischaemic colitis.

Answer These are shown in Fig. 16.1. The most characteristic sign is 'thumb-printing' or scalloping of the barium column. This is the result of localized elevation of the mucosa by submucosal oedema and haemorrhages. This sign may develop within 48 hours and disappear shortly afterwards or remain for several weeks. The 'thumb prints' are larger and smoother than the 'cobble-stones' of Crohn's disease. Later in the course of the disease, depending upon its severity, these radiological signs disappear to be replaced by tubular narrowing of the colon together with sacculation.

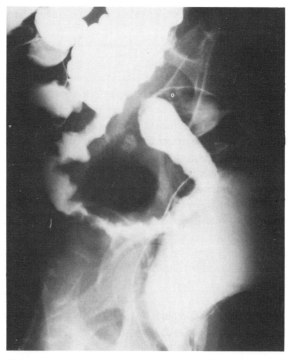

16.1

Question Which part of the colon is most commonly affected.

Answer The splenic flexure, transverse and descending parts of the colon.

Question Why should the splenic flexure be particularly susceptible to vascular damage.

Answer Because the blood supply to this area is frequently dependent upon a very small marginal artery formed by the inosculation of the superior and inferior mesenteric systems. Note the work of Griffith (1956) who found no evidence to substantiate the existence of Sudeck's critical point which Sudeck described as lying between the areas of the colon supplied by the last sigmoid and the superior rectal arteries.

Question What are the histological changes in ischaemic colitis.

Answer The histological changes depend upon the time at which the affected bowel is examined. In the early stages the changes are those of an acute inflammatory response associated with intravascular thrombi, haemorrhages in all layers of the bowel wall, oedema and necrosis.

In resolving ischaemic colitis in ulcerated areas the mucosa may be replaced by granulation tissue within which a marked proliferation of fibroblasts may be present. A characteristic feature is the presence of many macrophages filled with haemosiderin.

Question What would you consider to be the correct surgical procedure in this case.

Answer It is impossible to give a dogmatic answer. The following options are available:

1 Excise the affected segment of bowel bringing the proximal end of the bowel onto the surface as an end colostomy and closing the bowel distally.

2 Perform a transverse colostomy proximal to the lesion, leave the bowel *in situ* but drain the most badly affected area.

Comment Following either of these procedures the surgeon would anticipate the following:

Option 1: reopening the abdomen and restoring intestinal continuity.

Option 2: reopening the abdomen, excising the affected bowel and restoring continuity.

Primary excision and immediate anastomosis is *not* recommended in this condition because of the difficulty of defining the exact margins of the lesion.

In this patient the condition was complicated by her obesity and the presence of quite severe diverticular disease in the sigmoid. Option 2 was, therefore, adopted and the patient made an uninterrupted recovery, being discharged 16 days later.

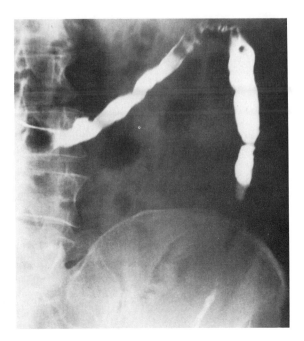

16.2

She was seen some six weeks later when a barium enema was ordered (Fig. 16.2).

Question What does this show.

Answer A long ischaemic stricture

Comment The patient was managing the colostomy well and refused to contemplate further surgery. She has, therefore, been followed up for some 12 years during which period she has developed symptoms of cervical spondylosis and required a cholecystectomy for intermittent but severe biliary colic.

17

A male, aged 61, was admitted complaining of intermittent peri-umbilical pain of six months duration. Each attack had been associated with severe vomiting, diarrhoea and abdominal distension and each had been increasingly severe. Throughout this period he had also noted an aching sensation in the right iliac fossa which had become increasingly severe and more persistent in the month prior to his attendance. He had lost 4 kg in weight in three months but disclaimed any loss of appetite.

Previous medical history Ménière's disease, first diagnosed 10 years prior to admission.

Physical examination There were no abnormal physical signs in any system.

Question What diagnosis is suggested by this history.

Answer The history suggests intermittent attacks of subacute small bowel colic.

Question Is the presence of pain in the right iliac fossa significant.

Answer It may be indicative of a lesion in the right iliac fossa. In view of the site of the colic and the progressive worsening of the attacks it suggests the presence of a lesion situated in the caecum which is obstructing the ileo-caecal valve.

Question What is the commonest mode of presentation of a caecal carcinoma.

Answer General physical deterioration associated with weight loss and anaemia.

Question How common is acute obstruction in the presence of right sided colonic tumours.

Answer Approximately 30 per cent of tumours situated in the caecum, ascending colon and caecum, as compared to 40 per cent of tumours situated in the splenic flexure, descending colon and sigmoid present with acute intestinal obstruction.

Question Why then does acute obstruction, due to right-sided colonic growths, appear to be relatively rare.

Answer Because tumours of the right colon are only half as common as tumours situated in the descending colon.

Question What investigations would you perform on this patient.

Answer
1 Double contrast barium enema.
2 Full blood count.
3 Ultrasonography of the liver.

Comment The results of the double contrast barium enema are shown in Fig. 17.1.

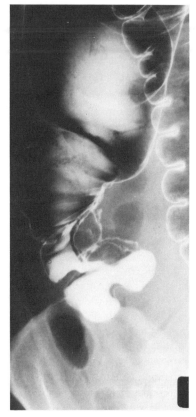

17.1

Question What does Fig. 17.1 show.

Answer The X-ray seen in the figure shows an abnormality in the caecum in which an asymetrically placed filling defect is evident arising from the ileocaecal region. The lesion is associated with mucosal destruction and the appearances are in keeping with a neoplasm. Note: no flow has occurred into the terminal ileum, a finding suggesting that the lesion is obstructing the ileocaecal valve.

Comment The full blood count was normal and ultrasonography of the liver revealed no change in the texture of liver.

Question What treatment would you advise.

Answer Right hemicolectomy following suitable bowel preparation.

Question What are the aims and methods of bowel preparation.

Answer Bowel preparation has two major aims:

1 The production of a colon-free from faeces.

2 The production of a colon in which bacterial colonization is reduced to a minimum.

The first aim can be achieved by a variety of methods which include:

(a) The administration of purgatives together with washouts and enemata. Common purgatives used include castor oil 60 ml and sodium picosulphate (Picolax, Nordic UK). The dose of the latter is one sachet containing 10 mg of the drug plus various additives taken at 08.00 hours and repeated at 14.00 hours and 16.00 hours on the same day, the contents of each sachet being dissolved in 30 ml of water. Whichever drug is used it should be given on two successive days prior to surgery following which a colon washout can be given.

(b) Whole gut irrigation. This was introduced in the early part of the 1970s and takes the form of a rapid flushing of the whole intestinal tract by irrigation from above. This method involves the passage of a relatively fine bore nasogastric tube through which is introduced a solution containing 6.14 g sodium chloride, 0.75 g potassium chloride, 2.94 g sodium bicarbonate per litre. The solution is warmed to 37°C and introduced at a rate of 75 ml/min. The first bowel action normally occurs within one hour and after clear fluid is passed the irrigation is continued for a further one hour. A total of between 9 and 15 litres of irrigation fluid is required.

However, the method is contraindicated in elderly patients suffering from cardiac disease since fluid absorption amounting to 1.5 litres may occur. It should also be used with caution in patients suffering from obstructive lesions of the colon.

(c) One litre of 10 per cent mannitol orally will provoke a profuse catharsis within 4–6 hours. Nausea can be reduced by the simultaneous administration of 10 mg of metaclopramide. Three disadvantages of this method have, however, become apparent: (i) a fall in plasma volume occurs which may be sufficient to produce a fall in blood pressure; (ii) a high count of gas producing *Escherichia coli* leads to the hazard of explosion if diathermy is used; (iii) a somewhat higher incidence of wound infection has been reported, chiefly due to *E. coli.*

The second aim is to decrease the colon bacterial count in order to promote better healing of the intestinal anastomosis and reduce the frequency of wound infection. It was not until the early 1970s that the importance of the anaerobic organisms, in particular, *Bacteriodes fragilis* was recognized as a cause of wound infection. A suitable antibiotic regime used by the author is as follows:

1 Neomycin 1 g. 12, 5 and 1 hour pre-operatively by mouth.

2 Metronidazole, 400 mg. 12, 5 and 1 hour pre-operatively by mouth.

3 Cephradine, 500 mg by intramuscular injection, one hour pre-operatively.

Question What is neomycin and what is its antimicrobial action.

Answer Neomycin is a bacteriocidal aminoglycoside effective against staphylococci, *Streptococcus faecales*, and a wide range of gram negative bacteria including *Escherichia coli*.

Question What are the contraindications to the use of neomycin.

Answer It is contraindicated in patients with a known history of allergy to the drug and it should be used with caution in patients receiving neuromuscular blocking agents, anticoagulants and other ·drugs which are known to be ototoxic.

Question In relation to colonic surgery what is the antimicrobial action of metronidazole.

Answer Metronidazole is a bacteriocidal agent which is active against *Bacteriodes fragilis* and *Fusobacterium spp.*

Comment Following bowel preparation an exploratory laparotomy was performed. This revealed a tumour of the caecum and a formal right hemicolectomy using an end to side anastomosis was performed. The tumour itself was mobile, the liver was free of palpable secondary tumour and only one palpable lymph node was present at the ileocaecal angle. The barium enema had shown severe diverticular disease in the lower sigmoid and this was confirmed.

Question What methods of restoring continuity of the gut after a right hemicolectomy have been described.

Answer Side to side, side of small bowel to end of colon and end of small bowel to end of colon.

Question In what circumstances is an end to end anastomosis most easily performed.

Answer In the presence of small bowel obstruction because in such circumstances the small·bowel will be dilated and its diameter will correspond more closely to that of the colon.

   If the small bowel is of normal diameter an end to end anastomosis is still possible if a cut back is made in the antimesenteric border of the terminal ileum.

Question What is the potential complication associated with a side to side anastomosis.

Answer A side to side anastomosis inevitably produces a blind end of ileum, this dilates and normally elongates with the passage of time and may eventually cause a 'blind loop syndrome'.

Question What is the essential feature of the blind loop syndrome.

Answer Malabsorption. This results from disturbed function of the gastrointestinal tract and causes an impairment of nutritional status together with a megaloblastic anaemia.

Question What is the cause of malabsorption following the formation of a blind loop.

Answer One known cause is bacterial proliferation in the blind loop. The large bowel is heavily colonized with anaerobic lacto-bacilli and gram negative coliforms and bacteriodes. When a blind loop is created as is inevitable in a side to side anastomosis stasis results in bacterial overgrowth. The results are:

1   Malabsorption of vitamin B_{12} due to bacterial competition for the dietary supply.

2   Impaired micelle formation and hence steatorrhoea occurs due to the disturbance of bile salt metabolism. Other unknown factors also play a part since treatment of this condition with an appropriate antibiotic may not necessarily alleviate the condition although surgical correction of the anatomical deformity is nearly always successful.

Question What are the characteristic clinical features of an exceedingly fatty stool.

Answer They are exceedingly foul smelling and greasy and float on water.

Question Why do fatty stools float.

Answer Because of the gas content rather than the concentration of fat.

Questions How is the degree of steatorrhoea quantified.

Answer By estimating the faecal fat concentration over a given period.

Question How is this achieved.

Answer The stools are collected over a given period the beginning and end of which is marked either by the oral administration of charcoal or carmine red or by a continuous marker such as chromium oxide or barium sulphate. When 1 g of the latter is given per day and the subsequent collection contains 4 g it can be safely assumed that a true four day collection of faeces has been made.

Question What is the upper normal value of faecal fat.

Answer On a diet containing 150 g of fat, 6 g/day.

Question What type of stitch would you use to complete the anastomosis.

Answer Either a two layer anastomosis or a one layer inverting suture technique can be used.

Question What is the anticipated incidence of suture line dehiscence.

Answer Between 5 and 10 per cent for anastomoses proximal to the mid-rectum.

Question What major factors govern the rate of suture line dehiscence.

Answer

1 Gross faecal leading.

2 Low pre-operative albumin.

3 Advanced age.

4 Site of anastomosis, anastomoses below the mid-rectum have a higher incidence than anastomoses at any other site.

Comment The following is the histological report on the resected tumour: this is a carcinoid tumour of the caecum infiltrating the ileum within the muscularis propria. Within the caecum the tumour has penetrated the wall of the gut and reached the periserosal fat. The tumour is of tubo-acinar pattern. A type C carcinoid containing PAS positive mucin within the alveoli. This tumour is argentaffin and argyrophil negative. Three of the six lymph nodes examined are invaded by tumour.

Question What stage as classified by Duke is this tumour.

Answer Stage C, see Viva 20.

Question When were carcinoid tumours first recognized and distinguished from adenocarcinoma.

Answer In 1928 as a result of the work of Mason.

Question What are the histological types of carcinoid tumour.

Answer There are three histological types of carcinoid:

1 The commonest type is the typical argentaffin carcinoid.

2 The non-argentaffin tumour.

3 The mucinous or goblet cell carcinoid.

The last of the group, i.e. type 3, has only been recently recognized and distinguished from adenocarcinoma. This type is composed of small clumps of cells distended with mucin which thus resemble normal goblet or signet ring cells. It was thought originally that this histological type did not occur elsewhere than in the appendix.

Question To what system do carcinoid tumours belong.

Answer The APUD system.

Question What is the derivation of this term.

Answer The cells of this system have in common the ability to secrete a polypeptide hormone and some also decarboxylate amine precursors to produce and store biogenic amines; in the belief that they all possessed this property they were called APUD cells, amine precursor uptake and decarboxylation cells. It is probably preferable to call them endocrine cells.

Question What secretions have been identified.

Answer Enteroglucagon, motilin, vasoactive intestinal peptide (VIP) gastro-inhibitory polypeptide (GIP), secretin and 5-hydrotryptamine (serotonin).

Question When was the endocrine potential of carcinoid tumours identified.

Answer In 1953 by Lembeck who found that carcinoid tumours may contain large quantities of 5-HT.

Question What is the normal distinguishing feature of the carcinoid tumours.

Answer Characteristically the cells of carcinoid tumours contain granules which are revealed by silver stains to which a reducing agent is added.

Question How is a cell capable of secreting 5-hydroxytryptamine identified.

Answer Cells containing 5-HT can be identified histochemically following aldehyde fixation since aldehyde together with 5-HT combine chemically to form β-carbolene which is fluorescent and acts as a reducing agent so that silver solutions attached to the granules are reduced; the argentaffin reaction. This complex also couples with diazonium salts to produce insoluble coloured azo-dyes, the diazo reaction.

Question What are the common modes of presentation of carcinoid tumours.

Answer

1 Within the appendix, acute appendicitis.

2 In the small bowel, intestinal obstruction.

3 As in this case, developing at the ileocaecal junction, intestinal obstruction.

4 Intussusception.

5 Hepatomegaly.

6 By producing excessive quantities of 5-HT causing the carcinoid syndrome.

Question What are the clinical features of normally active carcinoid tumours.

Answer

1 Flushing associated with a chronic cyanotic hue over the blush area.

2 Diarrhoea.

3 Bronchial constriction.

4 Heart failure due to the development of cardiac lesions. The

characteristic flush may be provoked by anger, mental tension, food or alcohol.

Question When do these symptoms become manifest in actively secreting tumours.

Answer When hepatic metastases are present.

Question What cutaneous lesions are associated with the carcinoid syndrome.

Answer Telangiectasia of the skin over the cheeks and the bridge of the nose.

Question What are the characteristic cardiac lesions.

Answer The cardiac lesions are highly specific. They are confined to the endocardium on the right side of the heart. In this region, on the valve leaflets and on the chordae tendiniae collagenous deposits develop. These last may cause valve stenosis or incompetence. The myocardium is separated from the fibrotic process by the internal elastic membrane which remains intact.

Question What rare deficiency syndrome may occur in patients suffering from the carcinoid syndrome.

Answer When large deposits are present in the liver more than half the dietary tryptophan may be converted into serotonin thereby diverting this aminoacid from niacin and protein formation. Thus patients may develop hypoalbuminaemia and pellagra.

Question What is the screening test for active carcinoid tumours.

Answer Estimation of the concentration of 5-hydroxyindole acetic acid in the urine. This is the major breakdown product of serotonin. The normal range is less than 58 mmol per day (11 mg per day). A false positive result may occasionally occur in patients to whom phenothiazines are being administered or who have eaten foods such as bananas or walnuts. A proprietary cough medicine containing glyceryl quaiacolate will also increase the amount of 5-HAA in the urine.

Comment Following operation the temperature and pulse rate are shown in Fig. 17.2.

Question In view of the intermittent pyrexia continuing from the first post-operative day what complication would you suspect and what investigations might be of assistance.

Answer The initial fever occurring 48 hours after operation could have been produced by massive pulmonary collapse, followed by infection of the affected segment. However, the continuation of the fever beyond this point suggests an anastomostic dehiscence with local abscess formation.

162

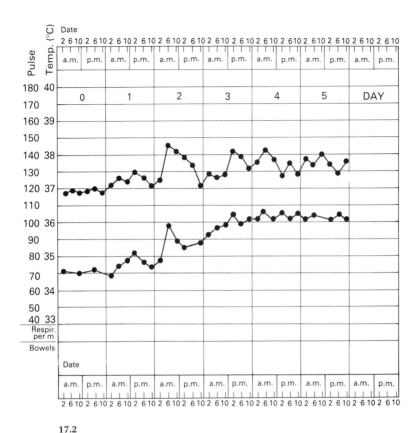

17.2

Question What physical signs are associated with massive pulmonary collape.

Answer The chief physical signs are as follows:

Inspection: Diminished movement on the affected side of the chest, tachypnoea and cyanosis.

Palpation: May reveal deviation of the trachea to the side of the collapse.

Percussion: Dullness to percussion over the affected lobe.

Auscultation: Diminished or absent breath sounds associated with crepitations at the edge of the affected area.

Question What are the chief radiological signs associated with massive pulmonary collapse.

Answer

1 A local area of radiodensity with increased lucency throughout the remainder of the lung fields.

163

2 Displacement of the interlobar fissures. When a lower lobe collapses the oblique fissures (Fig. 17.3), which in a lateral chest X-ray runs from the level of the third thoracic spine obliquely downwards and forwards towards the sixth costochondral junction, swings both downwards and backwards. This displacement is most easily seen on lateral X-rays. A lateral X-ray is very essential when the physical signs are on the left side of the chest.

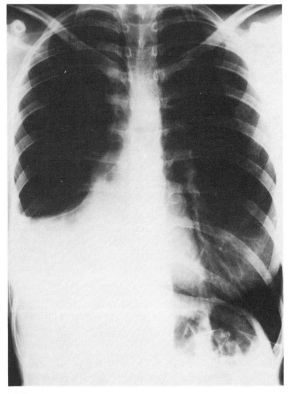

17.3

When the upper lobe collapses (Fig. 17.4), a much rarer event, in the PA projection the horizontal fissure is drawn upwards, becoming curved with the concavity pointing inferiorly.

Question What are the principle methods used for the treatment of pulmonary collapse.

Answer

1 Active physiotherapy including, if necessary, aspiration of the bronchial tree by endobronchial catheters. Such treatment is made

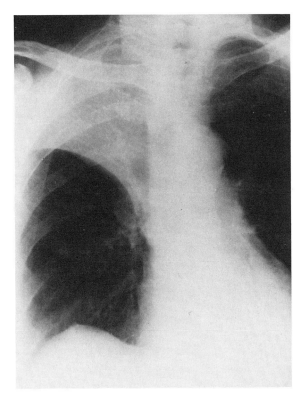

17.4

easier and more effective if adequate analgesia is administered prior to treatment.

2 Bronchodilators, e.g. salbutamol.

3 Antibiotics. Prior to obtaining bacterial sensitivity ampicillin is the most appropriate antibiotic since it is active against both the *Streptococcus pneumoniae* and *Haemophilus influenzae*.

Question What is salbutamol.

Answer Salbutamol is a sympathomimetic agent with prominent bronchodilatory effects due to the fact that it has prominent beta adrenergic activity with a selective action on beta$_2$ receptors. Symptoms of overdosage include a fine tremor of the hands, palpitations and muscle cramps. It can be used intravenously but is more commonly used in aerosol form (Ventolin, Allen and Hanbury's).

Question What local physical signs might accompany dehiscence of the anastomosis.

Answer Assuming that the infection produced by the dehiscence is localized to a subhepatic position it would be reasonable to assume that tenderness, rebound rigidity and cutaneous hyperaesthesia would be present in the right upper quadrant of the abdomen. However, in this patient the chest X-ray was normal and no abnormal physical signs were present on abdominal examination.

Question In view of the continued pyrexia what further investigations would you require.

Answer

1 A full blood count paying particular attention to the total nucleated cell count and the percentage of polymorphonuclear leucocytes.

2 An ultrasound examination of the upper abdomen.

Comment The TNCC prior to operation was 8.3×10^9 and on the fourth post-operative day 19.3×10^9 reaching a maximum of 26×10^9 with the percentage of polymorphonuclear leucocytes rising to 93 per cent.

Question Does this confirm the presence of pus in the abdomen.
Answer Yes.

Comment The ultrasound covering the whole abdomen showed a subhepatic collection of fluid (? pus) in the subhepatic region and a collection of fluid in the pelvis.

Question What are the eponymous names of these areas.
Answer A subhepatic collection is a collection in Rutherford Morrison's pouch which is bounded by the liver above, the transverse colon and mesocolon inferiorly, the kidney posteriorly and the duodenum medially and the abdominal wall anteriorly.

The pelvic collection develops in the Pouch of Douglas.

Question Are physical signs normally present when abscess formation occurs at these sites.
Answer Yes. A subhepatic abscess normally causes a palpable mass felt below the liver and a pelvic abscess a mass palpable per rectum in both male and female and also per vagina in female.

Question What are the classical symptoms associated with a pelvic abscess.
Answer A pelvic abscess is normally associated with fever, diarrhoea, tenesmus and the passage of mucus. On physical inspection when a large abscess is present the anal sphincter becomes patulous.

Question What is the precise definition of a subphrenic abscess.
Answer Any abscess developing between the under surface of the diaphragm and the level of the transverse mesocolon.

Question What intraperitoneal spaces are present.

Answer The right supra and infrahepatic spaces, the left anterior infra-hepatic space and the left posterior infrahepatic space. This last corresponds to the lesser sac.

Question What is the commonest site in which subphrenic abscesses develop.

Answer The right suprahepatic space, approximately 70 per cent of all subphrenic abscesses develop in this space and approximately 70 per cent follow general peritonitis caused by acute appendicitis.

Question What is the natural history of a pelvic abscess.

Answer In the majority of patients a pelvic abscess is a self limiting condition, only a minority requiring surgical drainage. The majority resolve spontaneously and those that require drainage can normally be adequately dealt with via the rectum or in the female through the posterior wall of the vagina.

Comment Repeated ultrasound examination of the upper abdomen showed that the subhepatic collection remained despite a variety of antibiotics, furthermore the fever continued and the white blood count remained elevated.

Question What would you do.

Answer Reopen the abdomen through the old abdominal incision. This was done, a subhepatic collection of pus was found together with a disrupted anastomosis.

Question What would you do.

Answer There are two possibilities.

1 The anastomosis could be completely disrupted and the two ends separately brought out onto the surface of the abdomen and the wound drained. If this course is adopted a further operation would, of course, be necessary to restore continuity at a future date.

2 Since the anastomosis was originally constructed with the middle colic artery and vein intact despite the presence of sepsis a revision of the original anastomosis could be made removing the terminal portion of the ileum and a small portion of the transverse colon.

Comment In this patient the anastomosis was refashioned and the sub-hepatic space drained. A central venous line was inserted and the patient fed intravenously for 12 days. The drain was removed on the third day following which his recovery was uneventful.

18

A male aged 71 was admitted complaining of a discharging wound in the right iliac fossa. This had been present following an operation performed some two years previously at which time a transverse colostomy had been performed and a rubber drain inserted through a stab wound in the right iliac fossa. His concern was the considerable amount of faeculent and purulent discharge which was necessitating between five and six dressings daily.

Physical examination

Respiratory system Air entry poor throughout both lung fields. Scattered rhonchi and râles supported a diagnosis of chronic bronchitis and further questioning elicited a history of a productive cough of several years duration.

Abdominal examination Inspection revealed a double barrelled transverse colostomy placed slightly to the right of the midline. A paramedian incision was present to the left of the midline. A sinus was present at the site of McBurney's point which was discharging thick pus.

Previous history Five years before admission he had suffered from a deep vein thrombosis accompanied by swelling of the left leg following a fall from a horse. This had been treated with anticoagulants and no further difficulty had developed.

Two years prior to admission he had been admitted elsewhere with a history suggestive of a purulent peritonitis following perforation of the large bowel. This had been treated by laparotomy, transverse colostomy and a drain had been placed into the peritoneal cavity through the right iliac fossa.

Sixteen months prior to admission in the hope that the transverse colostomy and the fistula could be closed the paramedian wound had been reopened, unfortunately the operating surgeon had felt unable to continue his abdominal exploration due to the density of the intra-abdominal adhesive.

Question What are the commoner causes of perforation of the large bowel.

Answer

1 Diverticulitis.
2 Colonic neoplasia; perforation occurring at the site of the growth or if the lesion is obstructive at the site of stercoral ulceration.
3 Ischaemic bowel disease.
4 Toxic megacolon due to ulcerative colitis.
5 Crohn's colitis.

6 Volvulus of the caecum or sigmoid.

Question In view of the length of history what would be the most likely cause of this patient's colonic perforation.

Answer Diverticulitis.

Question Who is reputed to have first described the condition of diverticulosis.

Answer Cruvheilher in 1849, deriving the term from the latin, 'divertere,' to divert or turn aside.

Question What are diverticula of the colon.

Answer Herniated mucosal sacs that appear within or without the wall of the colon.

Question Define diverticulitis.

Answer Diverticulitis may be defined as inflammation of the diverticula, with or without involvement of the adjoining tissues in the bowel wall and the peritoneum in the immediate vicinity.

Question Where do the diverticula occur.

Answer Diverticula appear, arranged in rows, chiefly along the edges of the longitudinal muscle bands at points at which blood vessels penetrate the gut wall from without in.

Question What is the most common site.

Answer The sigmoid and descending colon.

Question Do diverticula ever occur in the rectum.

Answer No.

Question Can the whole colon be involved.

Answer Yes. Some authorities believe that localized diverticular disease and generalized diverticular disease represent two separate conditions. Ryan points out that in generalized disease there is no muscular abnormality, that large bowel symptoms are unusual and that inflammation and perforation are rare in such cases whereas in disease localized to the sigmoid, muscular hypertrophy is prominent and the condition frequently presents with symptoms of colicky abdominal pain, constipation or diarrhoea and possibly acute inflammation.

Question What is the most striking pathological feature of the sigmoid other than the presence of diverticula.

Answer The appearance of the taenia coli which appear thick and may have an almost cartilaginous consistency. In addition the circular muscle is also much thicker than normal and has a corrugated or concertina-like appearance.

Question What is known of the aetiology of diverticular disease.

Answer The incidence of diverticulosis appears to be related to dietary habits. Diverticular disease and its complications are rare in the native populations of Africa in whom the normal diet is rich in fibre content. Painter & Burkitt in 1971 wrote a paper in the *British Medical Journal* entitled, 'Diverticular disease; a deficiency disease of Western Civilisation,' implying that the deficiency was one of fibre intake. This is of some interest since Sprigg's & Marxer some 50 years earlier were claiming that the appropriate treatment of the symptomatic condition was a low fibre diet.

The work of Painter suggests that diverticula arise as the result of disordered motility within an affected segment of gut. Pressure studies by this investigator revealed no differences between the normal bowel and areas of the sigmoid in which diverticula were present. However, when morphine was administered much greater increases in intracolonic pressure were recorded in areas affected by diverticular disease, the gut undergoing segmentation. It was within these zones of segmentation that the diverticula made their appearance.

Question What is the frequency of colonic diverticula in the UK population.

Answer The condition is rare below the age of 40. Thereafter it occurs with increasing frequency until 75 per cent of the population over 80 years of age have diverticulosis. However, symptomatic disease only occurs in about 10 per cent of those affected.

Question What symptoms may occur in the uncomplicated disease.

Answer

1 Intermittent lower abdominal pain.

2 A feeling of distension.

3 Constipation or periods of diarrhoea, not associated with systemic disturbance.

Question What are the chief complications.

Answer

1 Acute inflammation; according to the site of the sigmoid loop and its length, the acute pain and abdominal tenderness associated with this condition may be wholly confined to the left iliac fossa. However, if the sigmoid loop is long and lies to the right of the midline the condition may be easily mistaken for acute appendicitis.

2 Acute inflammation complicated by local abscess formation. This results in the development of a mass in the left iliac fossa. A plain X-ray of the abdomen in such a patient may show:

(a) A soft tissue mass in the left iliac fossa.

(b) A gas-filled cavity containing a fluid level lying in the region of the left iliac fossa indicating the presence of an extrinsic abscess.

(c) Local distension of ileal loops lying in the left iliac fossa.

3 Acute inflammation complicated by the development of a suppurtive peritonitis or a faeculent peritonitis.

170

4   Acute intestinal obstruction, which may develop as an acute condition in severe acute inflammation or as a chronic condition due to the development of a fibrous stricture if repeated attacks of less virulent inflammation occur.

5   Fistula formation. The inflamed sigmoid may adhere to any adjacent viscus notably the bladder, vagina, uterus or abdominal wall leading to the development of a fistula.

6   Haemorrhage. The usual explanation for the colonic bleeding, which may be life threatening in the elderly, is that the blood comes from vessels in the base of diverticula which are not necessarily inflamed. This explanation is substantiated by the fact that the majority of patients admitted with a severe rectal haemorrhage are completely symptomless and may have no previous history of colonic disease. However, attention has recently been drawn to the fact that the majority of these patients are elderly and the possibility arises that the diverticulae are incidental and that the bleeding is arising from areas of angiodysplasia, a condition most commonly seen in the elderly.

Question What is the natural history of diverticular disease.

Answer Parks & Henderson reviewed 531 patients suffering from the disease or its complications. They found that in 25 per cent some form of surgery was performed and that of the remainder treated conservatively only 20 required surgery at a later date.

Kyle reviewed 206 patients of whom 135 were treated conservatively and 71 required an operation and of these 35 were treated by a colonic resection. Of the total, 18 patients died on the first admission, nine of peritonitis, 12 per cent subsequently died of colonic disease, 10 per cent continued to have mild intermittent symptoms and 44 per cent remained well and free from symptoms.

From these retrospective studies it would appear that the great majority of patients admitted with complications but who do not require immediate surgery are able to continue life with at the most only mild symptoms.

Question What treatment is recommended for those patients with symptomatic disease who do not require surgery.

Answer A high fibre diet. Various reports indicate that between 70–80 per cent of patients remain symptomless on this regime.

Question Presented with a patient suffering from perforated diverticulitis and general peritonitis what surgical procedure produces the best results.

Answer A survey of the literature suggests that as an immediate measure a Hartmann's procedure gives the best results. Furthermore, if the distal bowel can be brought out as a distal mucus fistula there is every hope that bowel continuity can be restored at a later date. This would possibly have been the preferable operation in this patient at the time of the initial admission.

Question What investigations would you perform on the patient described.

Answer It is important to establish the tract of the fistula and its point of entry into the colon. This can be done either by a barium enema or alternatively, by injecting a radio-opaque medium into the external opening on the abdominal wall. In this patient both methods were used. The results are shown in Figs 18.1 and 18.2.

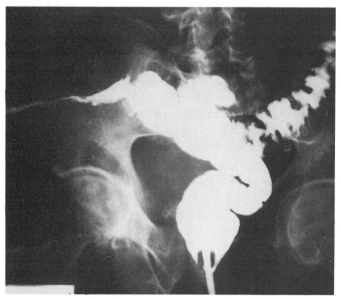

18.1

Question What do Figs 18.1 and 18.2 show.

Answer Figure 18.1 is a barium enema demonstrating a fistulous tract passing from the sigmoid colon towards the right iliac fossa. Diverticula and diverticulitis are seen in the descending colon.

Figure 18.2 shows the communicating tract from the right iliac fossa to the region of the sigmoid. Urografin has been injected through the external opening of the fistula.

Comment In assessing this man for operation we were particularly interested in his pulmonary function. In the course of investigating

172

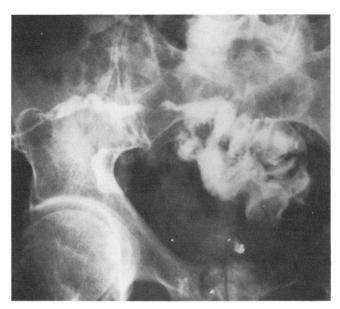

18.2

this a shadow was found on a plain X-ray of the chest. The appropriate tomogram of this area is shown in Fig. 18.3.

Question What does Fig. 18.3 show.
Answer A cavitating lesion consistent with a primary bronchial carcinoma.
Question What are the chief histological types of malignant lung tumour.
Answer
1 Squamous carcinoma.
2 Adenocarcinoma.
3 Small cell undifferentiated carcinoma.
4 Large cell undifferentiated carcinoma.
Question Does histological type bear any relationship to prognosis.
Answer Yes. When groups of tumours of comparable stage are compared differences in prognosis can be shown to be related to cell type.

As with the majority of tumours the better the differentiation the better the prognosis.
Question Which tumour has the best prognosis.
Answer Squamous carcinoma.
Question What percentage of tumours do not fit into this broad classification.

173

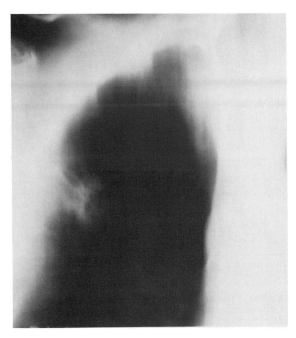

18.3

Answer Approximately 12 per cent. Some tumours defy histological classification, others are mixed adenosquamous, carcinoid or atypical
carcinoid.

Question Can staging be employed for bronchogenic carcinoma.

Answer Yes. The following is the TNM classification.

TIO   No evidence of primary tumour.

Tx   Malignant cells present in the bronchopulmonary secretions
but no tumour is visualized on plain X-ray of the chest or at
bronchoscopy.

TIS   Carcinoma *in situ*.

T_1 A tumour 3 cm or less in diameter surrounded by lung tissue
or the visceral pleura without evidence of invasion proximal
to a lobar bronchus at bronchoscopy.

T_2 A tumour 3 cm or more in its greatest diameter or invading
the visceral pleura, or, with associated atelectasis or accompanied by obstructive pneumonitis.

At bronchoscopy the proximal extent of demonstrable
tumour is within a lobar bronchus or at least 2 cm distal to the
carina. Any associated atelectasis or pneumonitis must

174

involve less than the entire lung and no pleural effusion is present.

T$_3$ A tumour of any size accompanied by extension into adjacent structures.

No   No nodal involvement present.

N1   Peribronchial or ipsilateral hilar nodes or both involved.

N2   Mediastinal nodal involvement present.

Mo   No known distant metastases.

M1   Distant metastases present.

Stage I is therefore composed of the following tumours:

T$_1$. No. Mo ⎫
T$_1$. N1. Mo ⎬ operable
T$_2$. No. Mo ⎭

Stage II

T$_2$. N1. Mo}operable

Stage III

T$_3$. any N or M stage ⎫
N^2. any T or M stage ⎬ inoperable
M1. any T or N stage ⎭

Question What are the chief diagnostic and staging methods used for bronchogenic carcinoma.

Answer

1   Plain X-ray of the chest with, if necessary, tomography. The cavitation present on the tomograph is highly suggestive of a squamous cell carcinoma.

2   Bronchoscopy associated with examination of bronchial secretions obtained by aspiration or by biopsy. Approximately 40 per cent of bronchogenic tumours are visible at bronchoscopy at the time of their initial presentation.

3   Computerized axial tomography.

4   Cervical mediastinoscopy or for left upper lesions, left anterior mediastinoscopy.

Question What are the chief modes of presentation of bronchogenic carcinoma.

Answer

1   A proportion are symptomless and discovered as in this patient as a result of a routine chest X-ray or alternatively, as part of a chest screening programme.

2   Haemoptysis.

3   Pleuritic pain, due either to an underlying pneumonitis or direct invasion of the pleura.

4   Unresolved pneumonia.

5   As a result of metastatic spread.

6 Rare manifestations include:

(a) Endocrine disturbances, chiefly due to the production of ACTH.

(b) Neurological manifestations, neuropathies combined with myopathy.

(c) Cutaneous disorders; dermatomyosites, scleroderma and acanthosis nigrans.

(d) Hypertrophic osteoarthropathy which may also be associated with Raynaud's phenomenon.

(e) Thrombophlebitis migrans.

Comment It was considered that the pulmonary tumour took precedence over the abdominal condition and after negative bronchoscopy but positive aspiration cytology the chest was explored through a right fifth rib thoracotomy. The lung was released extrapleurally with some difficulty, the visceral and parietal pleura being totally adherent due to inflammatory adhesions. The fissure between the right upper and middle lobes was developed easily and a right upper lobectomy was performed, the upper lobe bronchial stump being divided by an automatic stapler after which the line of division was reinforced with interrupted 4/0 sutures. No lymph nodes were identified.

Question Prior to closing the thoracotomy what test should be applied to satisfy the operator that the bronchial stump has been effectively closed.

Answer The stump should be put under forcible pressure by the anaesthetist, the thoracic cavity having been filled with water so that any escape of air can be easily detected.

Question What factors predispose to the development of a bronchopleural fistula.

Answer Ineffective closure of the bronchial stump but in addition the relative avascularity of the bronchus does not contribute to rapid healing.

Question Is an underwater drain necessary following lobectomy.

Answer Yes;

1 to drain any bleeding.

2 to remove air and allow the remaining lung to expand to fill the space left following resection.

Comment This patient made an uneventful recovery and in view of the subsequent histology, a squamous carcinoma; the small size of the tumour, 2.5 cm and the absence of nodal involvement the prognosis appeared to be good. A 40 per cent five year survival can confidently be expected in this situation. Therefore, six months later the patient was readmitted for further consideration of his abdominal condition. In view of the previous operative findings it was considered that it would be extremely difficult to excise the affected fistulous area of the colon followed by later closure of the transverse colostomy and that a possible alternative would be to perform a total colectomy excising the colostomy and performing an ileorectal anastomosis.

Question What bowel preparation would you advise.

Answer In an intact bowel one recommended regime is as follows:

2 litres of water together with 100 g of mannitol in 500 ml orally.

10 mg metoclopramide.

Neomycin. 1 g 12, 5 and 1 hour pre-operatively.

Metranidazole. 400 mg 12, 5 and 1 hour pre-operatively.

Cephradine. 500 mg by injection 1 hour pre-operatively.

Question What is the action of these various drugs.

Answer

1 Mannitol is an isomer of sorbitol. Normally administered by intravenous infusion as an osmotic diuretic it can be given by mouth to induce purgation. Given orally it may induce nausea and vomiting, hence the simultaneous administration of metoclopramide (Maxalon, Beecham).

2 Neomycin. This antibiotic is poorly absorbed from the alimentary tract, only 3 per cent of an oral dose being absorbed. The spectrum of antibacterial activity is similar to that of streptomycin sulphate. It is bactericidal and effective against the staphylococci and a wide range of gram negative organisms.

3 Metranidazole (Flagyl, May and Baker) is both antiprotozoal and anti-bacterial. Its importance so far as pre-operative preparation of the gut is concerned is in its action against the obligate anaerobes such as the *Bacteriodes* and *Fusobacterium spp.*

4 Cephradine (Velosef, Squibb) is a cephalosporin which acts like penicillin by inhibiting the synthesis of the bacterial cell wall. It is active against a large number of both gram negative and gram positive organism.

Comment Following the above intestinal preparation and adequate chest physiotherapy the old paramedian wound was reopened for the third time. As anticipated the whole of the small bowel was adherent not only to itself but also to the colon and the parietes. With great difficulty the various loops were separated, the colostomy limbs dissected from the abdominal wall and a total colectomy followed by an ileorectal anastomosis performed. The fistulous tract running from the sigmoid loop ran between various loops of small bowel and in separating the loops three tears were made in the small bowel, each of which was carefully closed in two layers. The total operating time was 4.5 hours. Three drains were left *in situ*, one in each paracolic gutter and one in the pelvis. Two units of blood were given during the course of the operation and this was followed by one litre of Hartmann's solution eight hourly intravenously.

Question What is the electrolyte composition of Hartmann's solution.
Answer Na^+ 130, K_4^+, Cl^- 109, HCO_3^- 28, Ca_3^{++} mmol/l.
Question What is the origin of the HCO_3^-.
Answer The HCO_3^- ion arises from the metabolism of sodium lactate.

Comment On the third post-operative day the urinary catheter was removed and the patient began to void spontaneously. However, on the fourth post-operative day following a bowel action the abdomen became distended, faeculent fluid began to discharge from the upper end of the wound, the blood pressure fell to 60 mmHg diastolic and the urine output diminished.

Question What events have occurred.
Answer
    1 Probably a leak has occurred either from the small gut torn at the time of operation but repaired or from the site of the ileo rectal anastomosis.
    2 Septic shock due to the liberation of intestinal contents into the peritoneal cavity.
Question What immediate action is required.
Answer The first essential is to deal with the septic shock. Usually following the administration of antibiotics one would consider opening the abdomen and draining the primary site of infection but since, in this patient, a fistula existed this seemed unreasonable. The patient was, therefore, placed on intravenous metronidazole and cephradine. In order to measure the urine output it was felt necessary to recatheterize the patient. This proved impossible with a silastic catheter but a simplastic coudé catheter was passed with ease.

    The general condition of the patient now improved but it soon became obvious that we were dealing with a high output fistula since between 1800–2000 ml of small bowel contents were discharged daily.

Question In the presence of a high output small bowel fistula what investigations and what treatment is required.

Answer

1 Repeated plasma and urine electrolyte concentrations.

2 Parenteral nutrition.

Question What is the chief indication for parenteral nutrition.

Answer Temporary intestinal failure. It is also possible using parenteral nutrition to maintain life in a patient with permanent intestinal failure, brought about by an extensive small bowel resection.

Question What are the commonest causes of temporary intestinal failure.

Answer

1 Small bowel resection prior to the development of compensatory changes.

2 High enterocutaneous fistula.

3 Severe complicated pancreatitis.

Question What are the general effects of a high output enterocutaneous fistula.

Answer

1 An inevitable loss of lean body mass which, if severe, i.e. above 30 per cent, leads to death.

2 A reduction in the immune response and, therefore, an increasing liability to infection.

3 Diminished wound healing.

Question What materials must be provided when maintaining a patient by intravenous nutrition.

Answer

1 An energy source. This can be provided by carbohydrate alone or by a mixture of carbohydrate and fat. Since there is a physiological maximum to the amount of glucose which can be oxidized in man some of the energy requirement is normally satisfied by the administration of fat. No more than 1600 kcals should be given as carbohydrate.

2 Amino acids, necessary for protein synthesis, 1 g N $\equiv$ 6.25 g protein $\equiv$ 25 g of muscle. In severely hypercatabolic states, as in this patient, the patient may lose 0.3–1.5 g N/kg per day $\equiv$ 2625 g of muscle tissue/day. During the convalescent period this requirement falls to between 0.1–0.3 g/kg per day.

3 Water. In order not to overload the patient carbohydrate is supplied as 10, 20 or 50 per cent solution and fat as an emulsion of between 10 and 20 per cent concentration.

4 Electrolytes.

5 Trace elements.

6 Vitamins.

Comment This patient was maintained by means of a peripheral line for eight days on the following daily regime. Freamine 500 ml: Novoplex, 1000 ml: glucose 5 per cent 2000 ml: trace elements, zinc 0.03 mmol, copper 0.015 mmol, manganese 0.018 mmol, chromium 0.4 mmol, iodide 0.1 mmol: intralipid 500 ml, heparin 1500 units and hydrocortisone 15 mg together with 10 ml of Multivite. On the ninth day a central line was inserted and intravenous feeding maintained for a further 12 days during which as the volume of fluid lost from the fistula declined, 500 ml of 50 per cent glucose was substituted for the weaker solution and the administration of both heparin and hydrocortisone ceased.

Question What is Freamine.

Answer Freamine is a proprietary aminoacid preparation manufactured by Boots. Each litre contains alanine 6 g, arginine 3.1 g, glycine 17 g, histidine 2.4 g, isoleucine 5.9 g, leucine 7.7 g, lysine acetate equivalent to lysine 6.2 g, methionine 4.5 g, phenylalanine 4.8 g, proline 9.5 g, serine 5 g, threonine 3.4 g, tryptophan 1.3 g, valine 5.6 g, sodium 10 mmol and phosphate 10 mmol.

Question What is Novoplex.

Answer Novoplex is a preparation containing the following: Na, 100 mmol; K 80 mmol; PO_4 38 mmol; Mg 7.5 mmol and 400 g of glucose per litre, thereby providing 1600 kcal/l.

Comment After stabilizing the patient an attempt was made to identify the site of the fistula. The most appropriate X-ray taken during the performance of a small bowel meal is shown in Fig. 18.4.

Question What does this show.

Answer A leak of the contrast medium through an irregular and complex tract into an adhesive bag. Contrast was also introduced per rectum which showed that the ileorectal anastomosis was intact and the conclusion reached was that the intestinal leak was probably arising from the ileum rather than the jejunum.

Comment On the fifteenth day the faecal discharge ceased and although a purulent discharge from the wound continued for a further fourteen days the patient was discharged approximately one month after his abdominal operation.

Three months later he presented in outpatients with a healed abdominal wound complaining of some difficulty of micturition. Rectal examination revealed moderate enlargement of the prostate, a fact already known from previous examination but the tissue removed on transurethral resection proved to be malignant.

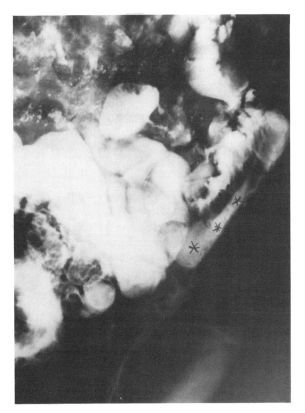

18.4

Question What is the incidence of carcinoma of the prostate.

Answer Approximately 6000 new cases are diagnosed per year in the
UK in which it is the sixth most common cancer. Between 15 and
25 per cent are diagnosed only after prostatectomy as in this case.

Question What diagnostic methods are currently used.

Answer

1   Rectal examination. The examining finger may detect a nodule
in the gland or in more advanced cases extra prostatic extension may
be present. However, of the many palpable nodules detected in the
prostate only 50 per cent will prove to be malignant. Therefore,
histopathological confirmation of the diagnosis is necessary.

2   Biopsy of a prostatic nodule can be performed via the perineum
or the rectum. If the rectal route is used a single dose of a broad
spectrum antibiotic should be given approximately 30 minutes before

181

the procedure in order to reduce the incidence of bacteraemia. This would be particularly important in an individual in whom any foreign material has been embedded, e.g. a prosthetic heart valve. In addition to confirming the diagnosis various histological features such as the pattern of cellular arrangement have been used as prognostic indicators.

3 Transurethral resection. This method of obtaining biopsy material is only used when the patient is complaining of obstructive symptoms.

4 Other methods used to stage the tumour as opposed to confirming the diagnosis include:

(a) computerized axial tomography.

(b) transrectal ultrasonography.

Question What is the TNM classification of prostatic cancer.

Answer T category T0, incidental carcinoma.

T1, intracapsular nodule, normal gland.

T2, intracapsular nodule deforming the gland.

T3, extension of the tumour beyond the gland.

T4, tumour fixed to neighbouring organs.

N category N0, no evidence of regional lymph node involvement.

N1, single homolateral regional node.

N2, Contra- or bilateral or multiple regional node involvement.

N3, Fixed regional nodes.

N4, Juxtaregional nodes.

In order to establish this category pedal lymphography would be required but this has a very significant error, as high as 30 per cent false positive and negative results being reported.

M0, no evidence of metastases, as judged by clinical examination, radiological and skeletal scanning.

M1, evidence of distant metastases.

Question What chemical marker is used in suspected carcinoma of the prostate.

Answer Serum acid phosphatase.

Comment This patient was treated by transurethral resection and remains well when seen one year later.

Question What adjuvant therapy has been practised for the treatment of carcinoma of the prostate.

Answer

1 Orchidectomy.

2 Stilboestrol, 1 mg tds. The adverse effects of this drug include

feminization, exacerbation of heart failure or hypertension, vascular complications, water retention, nausea and impotence.

Widely used following the initial studies by Huggins many urologists would now reserve this method of treatment for patients in whom symptomatic metastatic spread was present.

3 Progestogens. Medroxyprogesterone has been used but appears to have no significant advantage over stilboestrol.

Comment As with all endocrine manipulative methods although the initial response may be encouraging relapse occurs in the majority of patients within months. In all at least 30 per cent of patients show no evidence of any response whatsoever.

4 Chemotherapy. Cyclophosphamide, methotrexate and 5FU have been shown to produce some regression but their routine use is not recommended.

5 Radiotherapy. This is of proven value for the relief of bone pain.

If a patient fails to respond to oestrogens orchidectomy has nothing to offer and the reverse is equally true, oestrogens following orchidectomy have no value.

19

A male aged 55 years was admitted complaining of severe colicky lower abdominal pain. Although present for nearly two weeks the severity of the pain had markedly increased in the eight hours which preceded admission.

Previous medical history Eighteen months prior to admission this patient had been investigated for a complaint of intermittent abdominal pain of 25 years duration. He described each attack as colicky in nature, thus resembling the present attack but of less severity. Each attack had lasted between eight and 24 hours and was associated with gross abdominal distension and audible borborgymi. Normally the attacks terminated abruptly with the passage of a large volume of loose, watery foul smelling stool. The longest period between an attack had been one year and the shortest one month.

The investigations performed elsewhere, at a time when he was entirely symptom free, had included a barium enema, apparently demonstrating gross distension of the large bowel but no other specific features and a colonoscopy which was normal. A diagnosis of intermittent constipation was made and the patient reassured.

This patient had had no surgical interference.

Family history

1   One brother, a schizophrenic who had died of cancer of the colon some three years prior to the patient's admission.

2   One daughter, apparently operated upon at the age of 18 years for 'volvulus'.

3   One son who at 15 years of age had received surgical treatment for bladder neck obstruction.

Physical examination This revealed a large rather obese middle aged man.

Cardiovascular system	No abnormality, BP 120/70. PR 120, in particular there was no clinical evidence of dehydration.
Respiratory system	No abnormality.
Central nervous system	No abnormality.
Urinary tract	On direct questioning he admitted to some recent hesitancy but denied any diminution in the strength of his stream.
Abdomen	Inspection: gross generalized abdominal distension. Percussion: whole abdomen tympanitic. Auscultation: hyperactive, obstructive type of bowel sounds. Palpation: no masses palpable. Tenderness over the

whole abdomen with rebound tenderness in the right iliac fossa. PR: No abnormality detected.

Question What does this history suggest.

Answer Intermittent intestinal obstruction.

Question What are the common causes of intermittent obstruction which has apparently occurred over a period of 25 years.

Answer

1   In a patient who, prior to the onset of the attacks had a previous history of surgery, particularly if this had been complicated by intra-abdominal sepsis a diagnosis of intra-abdominal adhesions or bands would be reasonable.

2   In the absence of previous surgery intermittent volvulus must be suspected.

Question In a man of 55 would carcinoma of the colon enter the diagnosis.

Answer Not in this patient but certainly if the history had been relatively short and progressive.

Question Do the physical signs suggest a simple or strangulating type of obstruction.

Answer The presence of rebound tenderness in the right lower quadrant suggests the presence of a strangulating obstruction. However, objective analysis of large series of patients suffering from intestinal obstruction suggests that simple and strangulating obstruction cannot be distinguished with certainty on clinical grounds, particularly in the early stages.

Question What investigations would you order.

Answer

1   Full blood count.

2   Electrolyte values.

3   Plain X-rays of the abdomen in the supine and erect positions.

Question What might the full blood count reveal.

Answer It may reveal an increase in the haemocrit if haemoconcentration has occurred or alternatively, a fall in the erythrocyte count if a large strangulated segment of bowel is present.

Question Would you expect a leucocytosis.

Answer Yes. In both simple and strangulating obstruction a leucocytosis occurs in approximately 50 per cent of patients. In general the leucocytosis is greater, however, in patients suffering from a strangulating type of obstruction.

Comment In this patient the Hb and RBC count were both normal and the total nucleated cell count markedly raised.

Question What changes may occur in the electrolyte values in intestinal obstruction.

Answer Because distension of the affected bowel impairs the venous outflow to a greater degree than the arterial inflow the capillary pressure rises and diffusion of water and electrolyte occurs into the intercellular spaces causing intramural oedema which further impairs venous flow. As fluid accumulates iso-osmolar fluid with a sodium concentration approximately equal to that of plasma flows into the lumen of the gut. However, because the sodium concentration and the total osmotic pressure of the intestinal fluid is virtually identical to that of plasma this loss, by itself, will cause little change in the plasma sodium levels until the patient begins to vomit when the resultant loss of both sodium and water will result in clinical dehydration.

Changes in potassium concentration are also relatively late because of the large intracellular pool. A low potassium level, if present initially, is due to the clearance of potassium from the small extracellular pool more rapidly than it can be replaced by diffusion from the large intracellular reservoir.

Question What changes are present on the plain radiographs of this patient (Figs 19.1 and 19.2).

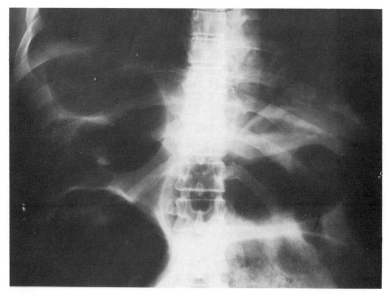

19.1

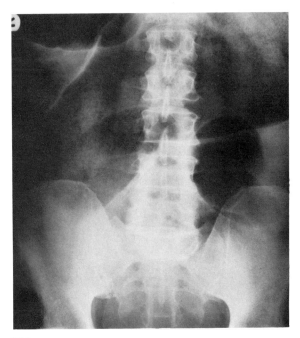

19.2

Answer Figure 19.1 shows a supine film of the upper abdomen. This patient was so large that the whole abdomen could not be exposed on a single film. This film suggests the presence of low small bowel obstruction because no valvulae coniventes typical of the jejunum can be seen. However, in the lower right hand area of the film an apparently distended loop of colon can be seen.

Figure 19.2 is a supine film of the lower abdomen showing further evidence of a distended gas filled loop of small bowel and confirms the presence of a huge distended loop of large bowel filled with faecal material which appears to be rising from the right lower quadrant.

Question What do these radiological signs suggest.

Answer The conclusion reached was that the patient was suffering from a recurrent caecal volvulus.

Figure 19.3 shows the typical radiological features of a caecal volvulus which are:

1 Great distension of the caecum which characteristically tends to migrate to the left upper quadrant.

2 Distended small bowel located to the right of the distended caecum, clearly shown in Fig. 19.2.

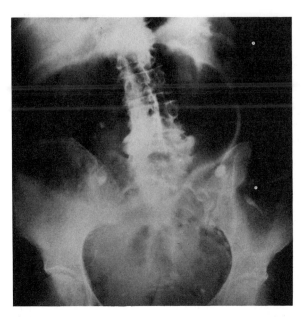

19.3

Comment The film presented was taken in the supine position and, therefore, no fluid level is present. However, migration of the caecum has occurred in an upperward direction from the pelvis and gas can be clearly seen in the descending colon.

Figure 19.4 shows the typical radiological features of sigmoid volvulus which are:
1 The greatly distended sigmoid loop.
2 'Looping' of the gas shadow to produce the typical 'bent inner tube' sign.

Question Is caecal volvulus more common than sigmoid.

Answer No. Caecal volvulus is considerably less common than volvulus of the sigmoid. The term caecal volvulus is a misnomer since in the majority of cases the terminal ileum and the ascending colon are also involved. Torsion occurs in a clockwise direction and may vary from 90 degrees to several complete twists. As with sigmoid volvulus there is, in the majority of patients, a previous history of recurrent attacks of abdominal pain which have spontaneously resolved.

Comment Six hours after admission this patient complained of even more severe abdominal pain. General examination at this time disclosed

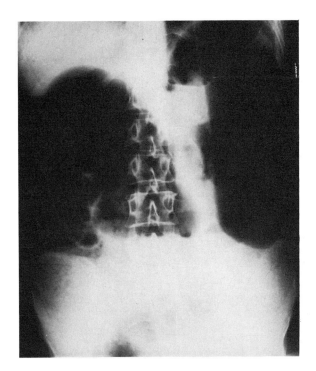

19.4

a pallid facies covered in visible sweat. His BP had fallen to 90/60 mmHg and abdominal examination revealed that the degree of distension had increased and that the rebound tenderness previously noted on the right side of the abdomen had increased in area and severity.

Question What might explain the rapid deterioration of the patient's condition.

Answer

1 Possible perforation of the bowel.

2 Toxaemia.

Question What is the aetiology of the toxaemia of strangulation.

Answer Probably both exotoxins and endotoxins liberated from a variety of aerobic and anaerobic organisms in the ischaemic gut.

Question How do these 'toxins' produce shock.

Answer By disruption of the microcirculation leading to a reduced circulatory blood volume and direct myocardial damage.

Comment The diagnosis of a caecal volvulus is an indication for an immediate operation and in this case following deterioration of the patient's general condition an exploratory laparotomy was performed immediately.

A catheter was inserted *per urethram* and left *in situ*. A right paramedian incision was made. This revealed a sigmoid volvulus, the sigmoid loop having twisted through 270°. In addition to the gross distension of the sigmoid the colon proximal to this was dilated as also was the small bowel.

Procedure The volvulus was rotated revealing a proximal constriction ring which appeared to be ischaemic. The sigmoid was then decompressed by passing a flatus tube via the anus into the grossly distended loop after which, following mobilization of the left colon, the sigmoid loop was resected and a two layer anastomosis performed between the distal descending colon and the rectosigmoid junction.

The patient received 500 mg of metronidazole intravenously during the course of the operation and 500 mg of Cephazolin intramuscularly one hour before surgery and at eight hourly intervals for five days.

The abdomen was closed with catgut and primary healing of the abdominal wound occurred.

Question If the correct pre-operative diagnosis had been made immediately following admission what would have been the optimum treatment.

Answer In 1947 Bruusgard recommended sigmoidoscopy followed by the passage of a flatus tube into the widely dilated sigmoid loop, the tube then being left in place for a period of 48 hours. This treatment has been successful in the author's hands on the two occasions on which he has attempted it. One feature of sigmoid volvulus which facilitates this technique is the gross hypertrophy of the sigmoid muscle which is said to make an extremely tight twist impossible.

A recently reported extension of this technique is reduction of the volvulus under direct vision using the gentle insufflation of air to visualize the point of torsion.

If either method is successful it can be expected that large volumes of flatus together with liquid faeces will be expelled. Thereafter an elective resection is required.

Question If the loop is already gangrenous when the abdomen is explored what surgical techniques might be considered to be more applicable to the situation.

Answer Either a Paul-Mickuliez type of procedure, leaving the patient with a double barrelled colostomy which can be subsequently closed or if the distal gut is gangrenous, Hartmann's operation bringing out the proximal colon as an end colostomy, closing the distal end and dropping into the pelvis.

Comment If a Hartmann procedure is performed later investigation will ascertain whether the continuity of the gut can be restored. Twenty-four hours after surgery the patient appeared much improved. His blood pressure had returned to normal levels 150/85 and his urine output via the catheter had reached an acceptable volume.

During the operative procedure he had received 500 ml of Haemaccel and 800 ml of plasma protein fraction. Following operation he received 1 litre of Hartmann's solution, 1 unit of whole blood, 1 litre of normal saline and 2 litres of 5 per cent dextrose.

Question What is plasma protein fraction.

Answer PPF is a sterile solution of the proteins of liquid human plasma containing albumin and globulins. It is prepared from pooled plasma from suitable human subjects, i.e. individuals in normal health considered to be free from transmissible disease such as syphilis, hepatitis B antigen and AIDS virus. Its pH is between 6.7 and 7.3, it contains not less than 4.3 per cent w/v of total protein and not more than 15 mmol (45 mEq) of citrate or 2 mmol (2 mEq) of potassium per litre. Ninety per cent of the protein is albumin and the remainder globulin.

Comment In view of the adequate urine output and the patient's denial of any serious voiding difficulties the catheter was removed after 48 hours. Over the following 24 hours he passed no urine and was, therefore, recatheterized 1 litre of urine being obtained. That night he became restless and demanded to be allowed to ring the neighbourhood policeman so that he could get rid of the Chinese dancers. It is of interest that unknown to us at that time he was studying Chinese.

Question What drug might be appropriate to control the agitation and hallucination.

Answer One drug which might be useful and was given to this patient is chlormethiazole edisylate (Heminevrin, Astra), which is a hypnotic and sedative. This drug is used in patients suffering from confusion, agitation and restlessness and in the treatment of alcohol withdrawal symptoms. Dose 750 mg in syrup, six hourly for two days, reduced thereafter.

Comment At the time it was thought due to the patient's occupation that he might be suffering from acute symptoms due to alcohol withdrawal. However, he later denied being other than a mild social drinker.

After recovery from his confusional state the urethral catheter was again removed. However, it soon became obvious that this patient was suffering from acute or chronic retention.

Question What would lead you to this diagnosis.

Answer Lack of any desire to void. After a period of 12 hours on an intake of 500 ml of fluid an hour he had no appreciation that his bladder was over distended and indeed after an intravenous pyelogram in which his catheter was again withdrawn recatheterization produced 2.5 litres of urine. A transurethral resection of his bladder neck was performed, minimal prostatic hypertrophy being evident either on rectal examination or on urethroscopy.

He voided on removal of the catheter in the third post-operative day and thereafter made an uninterrupted recovery.

20

A male aged 56 was admitted complaining of three months intermittent diarrhoea with the occasional passage of mucus and fresh blood. He had suffered no abdominal pain, no nausea or vomiting and lost no weight.

Previous medical history

1 49 years prior to admission he had suffered from rheumatic fever.

2 20 years previously he had suffered from pneumonia.

3 Seven years previously he had developed a right indirect inguinal hernia which had been treated surgically.

4 Six months prior to admission he had developed intermittent claudication in his left calf after walking a distance of approximately 100 yards.

Social history He was an extremely heavy smoker, smoking 60 cigarettes a day.

Physical examination

Respiratory system	NAD
Cardiovascular system	BP 140/90. Heart sounds—normal. Peripheral pulses, absent popliteal pulse on the left side and only weak anterior and posterior tibial pulses.
Abdominal examination	Negative.

Rectal examination revealed a large anterior rectal ulcer with raised edges.

Question What is the diagnosis.

Answer Rectal carcinoma.

Question What are the anatomical subdivisions of the rectum.

Answer The rectum is divided into three parts.

1 The lower third which extends 6 cm upwards from the ano-rectal junction, itself 3–4 cm from the anal verge.

2 The middle third extending from 6–11 cm.

3 The upper third extending from 11 to 15–16 cm.

Question Define the position of a rectosigmoid tumour.

Answer A rectosigmoid tumour is one which lies partly above and partly below the sacral promontory when the sigmoid loop is drawn out of the pelvis so that the upper rectum lies tautly along the front of the lumbo-sacral spine.

Question What is the frequency of carcinoma of the rectum in the various parts.

Answer Approximately one-third of all cases occur in each third of the rectum.

Question What investigation would you perform to confirm the diagnosis.

Answer Sigmoidoscopy and biopsy.

Question What is the value of sigmoidoscopy.

Answer It establishes the distance of the lower border of the tumour from the anorectal verge.

Question What is the importance of this distance.

Answer In the majority of cases it establishes whether a conservative sphincter saving operation is possible. It is generally agreed that tumours less than 5 cm from the ano-rectal margin can only be treated by abdomino-perineal resection.

Question Are there any exceptions to this rule.

Answer Local excision of small low rectal tumours, 3–4 cm in diameter, is recommended by many surgeons when:

1   The patient is unfit for a major surgical procedure.

2   The patient refuses to contemplate a colostomy.

3   The tumour is mobile on the underlying muscle coat, i.e. Duke's A stage tumour.

Question What is the value of biopsy.

Answer It confirms the diagnosis and by taking multiple biopsies establishes the overall degree of tumour differentiation.

Question What other symptoms may be present in a patient suffering from rectal carcinoma.

Answer

1   A relatively common symptom, absent in this patient, is an immediate desire to go to the toilet on waking in the morning. The 'explosive' motion then passed is composed chiefly of wind, mucus and blood.

2   Tenesmus, a constant desire to defaecate.

3   Pain on defaecation, normally only present when the growth has invaded the anal canal.

4   Pelvic pain, due to extra rectal spread, or sciatic pain from involvement of the sciatic plexus. When present this symptom indicates an extensive growth.

5   Symptoms associated with an ischiorectal abscess if perforation occurs.

6   Symptoms related to involvement of adjacent viscera especially the bladder or vagina.

Question What are the macroscopic types of established rectal carcinoma.

Answer

1   Polypoidal.

2   Ulcerative.

3 Annular.
4 Diffuse.
5 Colloidal.

Question What degrees of differentiation are recognized.

Answer Using Broder's classification four grades of malignancy are described, using Duke's only three. Low grade malignant tumours have the appearance of adenomata whereas high grade (Broder III and IV) consist of tumours in which there is no evidence of a glandular arrangement, many mitotic figures can be identified and there is evidence of deep vein invasion.

In addition to the above a colloid or mucoid tumour is recognized both macroscopically and histologically which cannot be satisfactorily graded.

Only a small proportion of rectal tumours are of low grade malignancy, nearly two-thirds are in the intermediate and highly de-differentiated grade.

Question How does carcinoma of the rectum spread.

Answer
1 By direct continuity through the bowel wall.
2 By extra mural lymphatics.
3 Transcoelonic.
4 Via the blood stream.

Question What is the importance of spread within the bowel wall.

Answer Spread within the bowel wall, in particular distal spread, frequently dictates the choice of the operation performed, i.e. conservative sphincter saving versus abdomino-perineal resection.

In 1913 Handley claimed that lymphatic permeation within the submucosa could be extensive and from this observation grew the conclusion that a clearance of at least 5 cm below the lower edge of the growth should be achieved. With the increasing desire of all surgeons to perform sphincter saving operations if at all possible Handley's concept has been repeatedly examined. The most recent data on this subject was that provided by Williams and Johnston in 1984 who found that in patients treated by abdomino-perineal resection in only 10 per cent had spread occurred more than 1 cm from the distal margin of the tumour and that in these patients the tumour was poorly differentiated and had already reached Duke's stage C.

Question How is carcinoma of the rectum staged.

Answer Rectal tumours are staged according to the extent of spread. The original classification was the staging proposed by Duke's (1932) who defined three stages, i.e.

Stage A. The tumour is confined to the rectal wall.

Stage B. The tumour has spread by direct continuity into the extrarectal tissues.

Stage C. Lymphatic metastases present.

The following modification of Duke's classification is also in common use:

Stage A. A tumour confined to the mucosa.

Stage B_1. A tumour extending to, but not through, the muscularis mucosa.

Stage B_2. A tumour extending through the muscularis mucosa with no involvement of the lymph nodes.

Stage C_1. A tumour limited to the wall of the bowel but with associated para-aortic lymph node involvement.

Stage C_2. A tumour limited to the wall of the bowel but with lymph node involvement extending to the highest point of the ligature.

Stage D. Local condition unimportant. Distant metastases present.

A number of modifications to Duke's original classification have been made, many of which merely serve to confuse the issue. In addition a complex TNM classification has also been evolved.

Question What is the relationship between the stage and ultimate prognosis.

Answer

1   When the tumour is confined to the submucosa 80 per cent of patients survive for five years.

2   When the tumour has penetrated the wall of the rectum, 45 per cent of patients survive for five years.

3   When lymph node involvement has already occurred 25 per cent of patients survive for five years.

Question What is the clinical significance of local fixity.

Answer The significance of local fixity depends on its cause, thus when the tumour is fixed by local inflammation it will have no effect on the prognosis but if the fixity is caused by malignant infiltration the prognosis is relatively poor.

Question In what proportion of patients is local spread already present at the time of surgical excision.

Answer Between 25 and 35 per cent according to the series examined.

Question Is the stage reached by the tumour at the time of diagnosis related to the degree of differentiation.

Answer In general the greater the degree of de-differentiation the more advanced will be the stage.

Question Can a rectal carcinoma be staged by clinical means alone.

Answer No. Even sophisticated staging procedures using computerized axial tomography do not give a true picture since involved lymph nodes, as opposed to enlarged lymph nodes, cannot be identified by this means. However, estimations of the carcinoembryonic and the acute phase reactant proteins can prove useful in discriminating between inflammatory and malignant fixation.

Recently a per-operative method of staging has been reported in which imprint cytology is used to examine nodes removed at the time of operation. The difficulty, however, is to find a lymph node in the mesorectum noting that Duke's staging depended upon the examination of every lymph node in the operative specimen. Imprint cytology in experienced hands normally gives rise to no false positive but may result in false negative results.

Question What is the incidence of synchronous tumours in colorectal carcinoma.

Answer Nine per cent.

Question What is the incidence of metachronous tumours.

Answer 2.5 per cent.

Question What is the anticipated presence of synchronous hepatic metastases in patients suffering from colorectal cancer.

Answer Approximately 20 per cent.

Question What is the influence of synchronous hepatic metastases on survival.

Answer The median survival time of patients presenting with a rectal tumour and hepatic metastases is 10.3 months. In a reported series this interval extended from 1 month to 4 years. The chief determinants of longevity are the degree of differentiation of the primary tumour and the degree of involvement of the liver at the time of surgery.

Question Is there a relationship between the incidence of metachronous tumours and adenomatous polyps.

Answer Yes.

Comment An abdomino-perineal resection was performed in this patient, after preparation of the bowel with manitol (20 per cent) 100 g orally together with three litres of water at the same time 10 mg of Maxolon was administered intramuscularly. Neomycin 1 g was given orally 12, 6 and 1 hour pre-operatively together with Metronidazole 400 mg at same time. The colostomy was fashioned by the extraperitoneal route. The tumour in this patient was 5 cm in length and 5 cm in breadth.

Question In a poor risk patient, is any alternative possible.

Answer Hartmann's operation which involves resecting the tumour with appropriate distal clearance and then closing the rectal stump. One advantage of this operation is the relative lack of 'shock' due to the absence of haemorrhage, the second advantage is that there is no perineal wound to heal.

Question Is there any advantage in practising high ligation of the inferior mesentery artery, i.e. ligating the artery at its origin in from the aorta rather than opposite the aortic bifurcation.

Answer Although seemingly more radical there is no statistical evidence of improved survival by this manoeuvre.

Comment The control of bleeding in this patient proved extremely difficult due chiefly to the small size of the pelvis. A further problem was the limited supply of blood, the patient being Group O Rhesus negative. Therefore, dissatisfied with the degree of control obtained a naked gauge peripack was inserted into the perineal wound and the perineal wound loosely closed around it. This was then removed after 48 hours with no recurrence of bleeding.

On the third post-operative day the patient passed flatus through his colostomy but on the fourth day he vomited.

Examination of the abdomen revealed slight distension and hyperactive bowel sounds.

On the fifth day he again passed flatus and a little motion through the colostomy but on the sixth day he vomited again. Examination now revealed marked upper abdominal distension and occasional exaggerated bowel sounds. However, despite this a little flatus was passed on the seventh post-operative day.

At no time did the patient complain of abdominal pain and there were no signs of an intraperitoneal infection, i.e. no fever or leucocytosis developed.

Question What is the diagnosis.

Answer This is the typical picture of incomplete small bowel obstruction.

Question How is it caused.

Answer The commonest cause following abdomino-perineal resection is the prolapse of a small bowel loop through the suture line of the pelvic floor, a less common cause is adherence of a small bowel loop to the small raw area distal to the extraperitoneal tunnel.

Comment After appropriate biochemical investigation the abdomen was opened through the original left paramedian incision and as antici- pated a partially obstructed ileal loop was found, not more than one-half the circumference of the small bowel having prolapsed through the reconstituted pelvic floor.

The loop, perfectly viable, was plucked out of the pelvis and the defect closed.

Question Give a brief historical account of the development of the synchronous combined abdomino-perineal technique.

Answer First suggested in the early part of this century by Bloodgood the operation was first abandoned and then revived by Devine in 1937 and by Lloyd Davies who in 1939 devised the adjustable leg rests allowing the patient to be placed and held in the Lithotomy-Trendelenberg position so that both the abdominal and perineal operators can work simultaneously without interfering with one another.

Question What innovative techniques have greatly increased the possibility of sphincter saving operations for tumours of the middle third of the rectum.

Answer

1   The development of the stapling gun. In using such apparatus the most important step is the insertion of the two purse string sutures which allow the colonic and rectal stumps to be tied in close approximation to the central shaft of the apparatus. A further important step is to examine the 'doughnuts' removed by the cutting blade which is held within the circumference of the staples. These discs or 'doughnuts' should be intact. If they are not it suggests that the anastomosis is incomplete and having identified the site the gap must be closed with Lembert sutures placed either from below, when the anastomosis is low or from above when it is at a higher level.

Question How would you identify the site of a leak.

Answer

(a) Instil methylene blue into the rectum. Not recommended.

(b) Fill the pelvis with saline and insufflate air into the rectum via a sigmoidoscope.

2   The development by Park's of abdominotransanal resection with a sutured coloanal or colorectal sleeve anastomosis.

In this type of operation the rectum is divided below a Parker-Keir crushing clamp which is closed some 2.5 cm distal to the lower edge of the tumour. A bivalve speculum is then placed in the anal canal and opened sufficiently to allow the submucosa to be injected with saline containing 1 in 200000 adrenaline. This injection floats the mucosa from the underlying internal sphincter and circular muscle of the lower rectum.

A cut is now made in the 'ballooned' mucosa 1 cm above the

pectinate line and the whole mucosal sleeve above this level is removed. The colon stump is then brought into view and sutured to the anal mucosal edge just above the pectinate line with interrupted 2/0 Dexon sutures, a bite of the internal sphincter being included in each stitch.

Comment The pathological report in this patient read as follows: an ulcerating, poorly differentiated tumour 5 cm in diameter involving the posterior quadrants of the rectum lying 3 cm above the pectinate line. The tumour is poorly differentiated and there is evidence of intra and extramural lymphatic involvement together with intra and extramural perineural involvement.

Eight lymph nodes are present in the specimen only two of which are involved.

The tumour was classified as Duke's C.

Question What immediate complication affects the perineal wound following an abdomino-perineal resection.

Answer Delay or failure to heal. This is due to a large variety of factors including:

1 The development of an hour glass construction at the level of the pelvic diaphragm or stenosis at the skin level. Both prevent the drainage of retained secretions.

2 Infection of the sacrum if the lower segment has been divided during the course of the perineal dissection.

3 Retention of foreign material.

4 The formation of a pilonidal lesion in the male.

5 Recurrent tumour.

Question What late complication of the perineal wound is occasionally seen.

Answer A perineal or sacral hernia. The author has only seen two during the course of his surgical career. The first occurred in a very elderly lady after the repair of a large paracolostomy hernia; the woman coughed whilst passing water and felt 'something giving way'. As she so succintly put it, she rose from the toilet with 'a monkey's bottom'. The second was the patient under discussion. A large variety of operations have been described to deal with this condition suggesting that no single operation meets with great success. The patient in question is symptom-free and his bulging perineum is supported by a pad.

Question What late complications may affect the perineal wound.

Answer Local recurrence. The incidence of local recurrence of a rectal cancer varies inversely with the height of the lesion and directly with the stage of the tumour. The highest incidence of local recurrence occurs with Stage C growths which involve the middle and lower thirds of the rectum. In these individuals local recurrence occurs in approximately one-third of all patients.

Question What is a phantom rectum.

Answer This syndrome is similar to that of the phantom limb after amputation, the patient having a sensation that the bowel is still present and that flatus and/or faeces are present.

Question What is the principle early complication affecting the colostomy.

Answer Necrosis followed by retraction.

Question What are the common late complications affecting the colostomy.

Answer

1 Stenosis, this normally follows necrosis.

2 Pericolostomy herniation.

3 Prolapse.

Question What disorders of sexual function may follow low anterior or abdominoperineal resection.

Answer

1 Damage to the parasympathetic may lead to impotence. In the author's experience this is much more likely to occur following the removal of growths restricted to the wall of the bowel in which neither inflammatory or neoplastic infiltration has occurred.

2 Failure of ejaculation due to damage to the sympathetic nervous system.

Question How frequent are these complications.

Answer Approximately one-third of patients, previously enjoying normal sexual function, will become impotent and approximately fifty per cent of these patients will fail to ejaculate.

Question What adjuvant therapy has been employed in the treatment of carcinoma of the rectum.

Answer

1 Pre- and post-operative deep X-ray therapy.

2 Chemotherapy.

Question Does either method of treatment confer benefit in terms of overall prognosis.

Answer So far as deep X-ray is concerned the question still remains open. So far as chemotherapy is concerned the most effective drug appears to be 5-Fluorouracil. Approximately 20 per cent of rectal tumours respond to this drug both *in vitro* and *in vivo* but various published series indicate that chemotherapy certainly does not delay the progression or prolong the survival of patients in whom local residual disease is known to be present following surgery.

Question What symptoms are associated with local pelvic recurrence or the extension of residual pelvic disease.

Answer The development of persistent perineal, sacral or sciatic pain and in some patients the gradual appearance of a swelling in the perineum which eventually ulcerates to produce a typical malignant ulcer.

Question What is the survival rate for patients treated surgically for carcinoma of the rectum.

Answer All stages: 57.4 per cent at five years falling to 49.8 per cent at 20 years. However, in Stage A a five year survival of 95 per cent can be expected compared to a 40 per cent survival after this interval for Stage C tumours.

21

A female aged 40 presented in surgical outpatients complaining of a painless swelling in the upper and outer quadrant of the right breast.

Question What physical signs would suggest a clinical diagnosis of malignancy.

Answer A solid swelling associated with any of the following physical signs; skin fixation, deep fixation, nipple displacement or retraction, general asymmetry of the breast, skin oedema (peau d'orange), satellite nodules in the skin, ulceration of the skin overlying the swelling, or palpable axillary lymph nodes.

Comment This swelling was approximately 1.5 cm in diameter and tethered to the overlying skin and a clinical diagnosis of malignancy was therefore made.

Question In the absence of the specific physical signs described what other condition might produce a solitary swelling in the breast in a female of this age.

Answer
1 A fibroadenoma.
2 A cyst.
3 Fat necrosis.

Question What clinical types of fibroadenoma are described.

Answer The hard and the soft. The former, usually occurring in young women is histologically described as a pericanalicular fibroadenoma but in a female of this age the more common type is the soft, or intracanalicular fibroadenoma. This tumour may grow to such a size that the skin overlying the swelling may undergo necrosis, an ulcer forms and the lesion mimicks a malignant condition. A malignant variant of this condition, cystosarcoma phyllodes, was described by Muller in 1938.

Question What is the frequency of breast cancer.

Answer Carcinoma of the breast is the commonest cancer in females. Six per cent of all women develop a cancer of the breast in their lifetime in contrast to a lifetime incidence of cancer overall of 27 per cent. Thus in one out of every four women suffering from cancer the primary site will be the breast.

Question In the light of clinical findings: what stage is this tumour.

Answer On the simple staging system, commonly referred to as the Manchester System, this tumour has reached Stage I.

Question What are the defined stages of the Manchester System.

Answer Stage I. A tumour is present in the breast which is 5 cm or less in diameter. If skin changes are present they are limited to the skin immediately overlying the tumour.

Stage II. The tumour is of identical dimensions to that found in Stage I but palpable mobile axillary lymph nodes are present.

Stage III. The tumour is larger than 5 cm in diameter and/or fixed axillary lymph nodes are present.

Stage IV. Regardless of the local condition distant metastases are already present.

Question What is the alternative staging system.

Answer The TNM classification developed by the Union Internationale Contre Cancer (UICC). This is an unwieldy system. For example, T, the tumour stage, is divisible into 10 subsets added to which a post-operative histopathological staging can also be applied. This system is, therefore, most frequently used in research projects in which specific but different treatments are being applied to randomized groups of patients.

Question What is fallacy with both staging methods.

Answer Neither take account of internal mammary lymph node involvement, which can only be established by performing an extended radical mastectomy or by biopsy performed at the time of less radical surgery.

There is also considerable observer variation particularly in regard to the size of the swelling and the presence or absence of enlargement of the axillary lymph nodes. In addition there is approximately a 33 per cent difference in the clinical and pathological evaluation of the axillary nodes.

Question What major risk factors have been identified by epidemiological study.

Answer

1 An early menarche.
2 A late first full term pregnancy.
3 Late menopause.
4 Post-menopausal weight.

Comment In this female, factors 1 and 2 were applicable. The menarche had occurred at 12 years of age and her first and only child was six years of age.

Question How accurate is clinical examination.

Answer In the presence of the above physical signs the diagnosis of malignancy is highly probable. However, fat necrosis may produce many of the physical signs described, e.g. skin tethering and palpable axillary nodes although in this condition there is frequently a history of severe bruising following an injury prior to the development of a swelling.

Question What is the importance of an accurate determination of nodal involvement.

Answer Nodal involvement markedly affects the prognosis. Thus:

1 Occult neoplastic involvement, i.e. nodal involvement discovered only on serial section has little or no influence on the prognosis.

2 Pathological involvement discovered without the need for serial section reduces the 5 and 10 year survival of the breast cancer patient to 52 and 32 per cent respectively.

3 The number of nodes involved is also important. When less than four nodes are pathologically involved a 10 year survival of 32 per cent may be anticipated whereas if four or more nodes are involved the survival rate falls to approximately 14 per cent.

Question In a patient presenting with a swelling of indeterminate physical nature what special investigations may be used apart from open biopsy and frozen section.

Answer

1 Mammography or xeroradiography.

2 Fine needle aspiration cytology.

3 Thermography, although this is seldom used.

Question What is the technical advantage of xeroradiography over mammography.

Answer The chief advantage is known as the 'edge enhancement effect'. This effect makes the boundaries of areas of uneven density, particularly easy to see. Thus calcification, rough edges and junctional lines are clearer. A disadvantage of xeroradiography is in the reproduction of unclear limited densities behind which a solid carcinoma may be hiding.

Question What are the chief mammographic features which suggest malignancy.

Answer

1 Calcifications.

2 Local increases in density within the breast.

3 Structural changes within the breast.

4 Indirect indications such as vascular signs.

Question In what proportion of breast cancers is calcification present on mammography.

Answer Approximately three-quarters.

Question Does calcification occur in benign lesions.

Answer Yes. However, the calcification occurring in benign tumours is usually extremely coarse or ring-like. In malignant disease micro-calcifications occur which consist of accumulations of calcium with amorphous, bizarre shapes which differ in size. The smallest of these calcific areas may be only 0.1 mm in diameter.

Question What structural changes indicating malignancy may be seen on a mammograph.

Answer Many breast carcinomata are associated with fibrosis, e.g. scir-rhous cancers. As such, fibrotic extensions radiate from the dense area produced by the tumour itself. Such radial extensions range from fine lines to wide pointed stripes which break through the natural pattern produced by the normal connective tissue.

Question What is the accuracy of mammographic as compared to clinical examinations.

Answer Mammography is more accurate than clinical examination in the diagnosis of lesions which are less than 2 cm in diameter. When the malignant lesion is 0.5 cm or less in size, i.e. barely discernable on clinical examination unless it is superficially placed in a small breast, mammography is some five times more accurate than simple clinical examination.

Question What is the overall accuracy of mammography.

Answer Between 85–95 per cent. False negative results are particularly common in pre-menopausal women in whom small tumours may cause no identifiable changes.

Question In what groups of women might routine mammography be particularly useful.

Answer In high risk patients, i.e. those in whom a close blood relation has suffered from the disease or when a cancer has already been removed from one breast.

Question What type of breast lesion can be investigated by fine needle aspiration cytology.

Answer Any palpable swelling which can be fixed between finger and thumb before the insertion of the needle.

Question How is this technique performed.

Answer A 22–23 gauge needle is fixed to a disposable syringe and under negative pressure the needle is passed several times through the swelling. After releasing the pressure the needle is withdrawn and removed from the syringe which is then refilled with air. The contents of the needle are then reinjected and smeared onto a glass slide. The smear is air dried and then stained.

Question What is the accuracy of aspiration cytology of the breast,

Answer As with any other investigation much depends upon the experi-ence of the cytologist. Experienced investigators in this field report false negative results of the order of 10 per cent and false positive results of the order of 0.1 per cent.

Comment Because of the lateral position of the swelling in this patient only the upper and outer quadrant of the breast was removed and the contents of the axilla sampled. The histology of the excised breast tissue showed the presence of an infiltrating ductal carcinoma, with involvement of the single lymph node found in the axillary fat.

Question What other histological types of breast cancer are recognized.

Answer Infiltrating ductal carcinoma comprise the commonest form of breast cancer. The less common types include:

1 Medullary carcinoma.
2 Infiltrating lobular carcinoma.
3 Mucinous (colloid) carcinoma.
4 Tubular carcinoma.
5 Papillary carcinoma.
6 Adenoid-cystic carcinoma.

Question What is meant by the term 'inflammatory carcinoma'.

Answer This is a purely clinical term which refers to a tumour accompanied by the symptoms of redness and warmth of the skin overlying the tumour. The histological basis for this appearance is dermal lymphatic carcinomatosis although this condition can present with peau d'orange without any clinical signs of inflammation.

Question Are breast tumours histologically homogenous.

Answer Not necessarily. Approximately one- third of all tumours are composed of more than one histological type. Even the cells of the tumour may behave differently when cultured *in vitro*. Thus differences in growth rate, differentiation, antigenicity, immunogenicity, chromosomal ploidy can all be demonstrated in cells from different parts of the same tumour. Recently it has also been found that different parts of the same tumour may have different concentrations of oestrogen receptors.

Question In view of clinical and pathological findings what is the tumour stage in this patient.

Answer On the simple Manchester Classification, Stage II, on the more complex TNM classification system T1a N1b Mo.

Question In view of the stage what are the statistical chances of this patient surviving 10 years.

Answer Approximately 40 per cent.

Question Can it ever be said that a patient suffering from carcinoma of the breast is cured.

Answer Probably not. The original statistical analysis of survival of patients suffering from breast cancer, followed for approximately 25 years by Brinkley and Haybittle, suggested that cure based on the definition of Easson and Russel (which was as follows: we may speak of cure of a disease when there remains a group of disease free survivors, probably a decade or two after treatment whose annual death rate from all causes is similar to that of the normal population group of the same age and sex distribution) was achieved if the patient survived for approximately 20 years following diagnosis and treatment. This opinion expressed by Brinkley and Haybittle was based on an analysis of some 704 breast cancer patients treated between the years 1947 and 1950. However, a recent analysis of the same group covering 30 years showed that despite the parallelism of the survival curves between the normal population and breast cancer patients at 20 years a further divergence occurred thereafter. One explanation for this somewhat unexpected result advanced by Brinkley and Haybittle was that the increased risk of death was in some way attributable to treatment and all that it involves.

Question What are the chief factors which influence survival in breast cancer patients.

Answer

  1 Lymph node status. When more than four axillary nodes are involved the chances of survival are greatly reduced. Although various figures have been produced the general statement that the number of axillary nodes involved is inversely proportional to the patient's survival holds good.

  2 Tumour size. Not only does the absolute size of the breast tumour appear to affect the prognosis in an individual case it also influences the chances of metastases. Thus the smaller the tumour the less frequent will be the presence of involved axillary nodes. The size of the tumour is directly related to the growth rate. Thus Gershon-Cohen and his associates showed in 1967 that the rate of breast tumour growth was very variable. They found that the doubling time of a breast tumour could vary between 23 and 209 days, the average being 100 days. The significance of this finding is that with a low doubling time it would take only two years for a tumour to reach 1 cm in size whereas when the doubling time was 200 days it would take some 17 years. However, it is highly probable that as a tumour increases in size the exponential growth pattern is lost because the decreased oxygen tension in the interior of the tumour causes necrosis.

  3 Histological grade. The grading of tumours is based on work

performed in the twenties by Greenough. Three grades were defined based on the degree of tubule formation, the size and shape of cells and nuclei and on the frequency of hyperchromasia and mitosis. Upon this basis Greenough subdivided mammary tumours into three grades: grade 1, well differentiated; grade 2, moderately differentiated; grade 3, undifferentiated. Although ignored for some three decades the method was revived by Bloom in 1956 who again showed that there was a close correlation between survival time and tumour grade. Since then there has been some argument as to whether general grading of the type described or nuclear grading is the more important. Nuclear grading is achieved by taking note of marked variations in the size and shape of the nuclei, the prominence of nucleoli, chromatin clumping and the frequency of mitotic figures. Thus tumour nuclei which are similar in size and in appearance to those in the normal breast tissue are defined as differentiated, the converse leading to the diagnosis of undifferentiated.

4 Oestrogen Receptor Status. Although Beatson in 1896 discovered that some breast tumours could be controlled, at least temporarily by oophorectomy, it was not until 1967 that Elwood Jensen and his colleagues produced a scientific explanation for this phenomenon.

They established that an important difference between hormone dependent and non-dependent tissues was the ability of oestrogen dependent tissues to concentrate oestradiol. This basic observation led to the discovery of intracellular oestrogen-binding components termed receptors which bound the steroid and were responsible for the concentration effect. It is now certain that in the breast cells the hormone, i.e. oestradiol, functions by becoming bound to cytoplasmic receptor protein. Once so bound the nuclear oestrogen receptor complex leads to the production of components essential for cell maintenance and function.

One of the chief problems associated with the measurement of the amount of oestrogen receptor present in breast tumour cells has been the difficulty of standardizing the methodology of measurement. At first it appeared that only tumour cells possessing oestrogen receptors were capable of responding to anti-oestrogen therapy and that oestrogen receptors were more commonly found in greatest concentration in well differentiated tumours. Both these hypotheses have now been disproved although a relationship exists between the amount of oestrogen receptor and the response to anti-oestrogens. Thus the NATO trial shows that high concentrations of oestrogen receptor are associated with prolonged survival when patients are treated with the anti-oestrogen, Tamoxifen (Nolvadex ICI).

Whilst oestrogen receptors have received most attention the importance of both progesterone and androgen receptors is now being appreciated.

5   Age. Patients less than 50 years of age have a significantly worse prognosis than women over the age of 50 whether considered overall or relative to their nodal status.

Question What markers other than oestrogen receptors occur in cancer of the breast.

Answer Various tumour related antigens, CEA, HCG and casein develop both in malignant and benign breast disease but they are of little practical use because although the frequency with which they occur increases with the tumour load they are not sufficiently sensitive to distinguish between malignant and benign breast disease.

Comment Following recovery from her segmental resection this patient was treated with radiotherapy to the breast, axilla and supraclavicular regions.

Question For radiotherapy to achieve maximal effect what is required.

Answer A well-oxygenated cell. Anoxic cells are resistant to the effects of irradiation.

Question Is there any evidence that radiotherapy prolongs survival.

Answer No. The purpose of radiotherapy is to control local disease, e.g. recurrence in the chest wall and so prolong the disease free interval.

Question Other than wide local excision of the tumour what other surgical operations have been described for the treatment of operable breast cancer.

Answer

1   Halsted's radical mastectomy. Halsted described this operation in 1894. The operation consists of removal of the breast, the pectoralis major and minor muscles and clearance of the axilla from the apex, the posterior boundary of the dissection being the anterior border of the latisimus dorsi muscle.

2   Total or simple mastectomy. This operation involves removal of the breast with a skin margin of at least 4 cm on either side of the tumour together with the axillary tail of Spence. Since no axillary dissection is performed this operation has been criticized on the grounds that no information is obtained regarding the involvement or otherwise of the axillary nodes.

3   Modified radical operation. In this operation the pectoralis major muscle is left intact but a dissection of the axilla is performed by dividing the attachment of the pectoralis minor to the coracoid process.

4   Extended or supraradical mastectomy. This operation, not

popular in the UK, consists of a radical mastectomy together with an en bloc excision of the internal mammary chain of nodes. The consensus opinion appears to be that survival is not improved by this extensive procedure.

Question What argument has been advanced against merely treating a breast cancer by local tumour excision.

Answer There is a substantial incidence of multifocal lesions in breast cancer patients involving both breasts. However, only rarely is there evidence of two or more overt lesions in the same breast and synchronous bilateral tumours are also uncommon. Furthermore the incidence of asynchronous primary tumours in the uninvolved breast fails to approach the incidence of occult lesions detected by random biopsy, evidence that not all cancers progress to overt lesions.

Comment Two years following her initial treatment this patient presented with a skin nodule in the scar. This was widely excised and proved to be malignant.

Question What does this suggest.

Answer That the tumour was relatively insensitive to irradiation.

Comment No further treatment was given and one year later the patient presented with a swelling within the breast tissue itself in immediate relationship to the site of the original tylectomy.

Question What would you advise.

Answer Mastectomy.

Comment This patient was now told that a mastectomy was indicated. This was performed, the axilla was explored but no palpable lymph nodes were discovered. Some six years later, however, i.e. nine years after her initial presentation, palpable lymph nodes developed in the axilla.

Question What treatment would you offer.

Answer A block dissection of the axilla.

Question What long-term complication might follow such treatment.

Answer Lymphoedema of the arm.

Question What is the incidence of this complication.

Answer Statistics vary but severe disabling lymphoedema is in the author's experience rare. However, some measurable difference in the circumference of the arm on the affected side is relatively common, being present in about one-third of all patients.

Comment At this time the anti-oestrogen Tamoxifen (Nolvadex ICI) had been placed on the market and the patient was prescribed 10 mg tds.

Question What is the action of Tamoxifen.

Answer A simplistic view of the action of Tamoxifen was advanced in 1975 when it was presumed that any benefit derived from this drug was the result of its binding to the oestrogen receptor and thus interfering with the action of oestradiol. However, more complex explanations have now been put forward.

Question What are the adverse effects of Tamoxifen.

Answer A variety of adverse effects have been reported including hot flushes, pruritis, dizziness and rashes but the great majority of patients tolerate this drug exceedingly well.

Comment The beneficial effect of Tamoxifen has now been demonstrated by the careful clinical trials organized by Imperial Chemical Industries plc. It has been found that this drug not only prolongs the disease-free interval but more importantly perhaps prolongs survival. These positive results are particularly evident when the tumour has high concentrations of oestrogen receptors.

Question What is meant by the term adjuvant therapy.

Answer Adjuvant therapy is therapy administered at the time of the initial surgical treatment. Radiotherapy can be regarded as adjuvant therapy but the term is more loosely applied to the administration of cytotoxic or hormonal therapy.

Question What is the rationale for the administration of cytotoxic agents.

Answer This has changed with the passage of time. Initially these agents were used in the hope that tumour cells liberated into the circulation at the time of the initial operation would be killed. It is now more common to administer repeated pulses of chemotherapy over a prolonged period post-operatively in the hope that micrometastases will be eliminated.

Question What cytotoxic drugs are commonly used.

Answer Thiotepa and phenylalanine mustard are commonly used as a single agent treatment and CMF, i.e. cyclophosphamide, methotrexate and 5-fluorouracil in combination. There remains some doubt as to the overall effectiveness of these drugs and in particular which subset of patients will benefit. Nissen Meyer believes that prolongation of the disease-free interval by cytotoxic agents is due to ovarian suppression in the pre-menopausal group whereas Bonnadonna of Milan now claims that there is no difference in the response achieved in pre-menopausal and post-menopausal women. He believes that previous results showing that adjuvant chemotherapy was of greater benefit in pre-menopausal women was due to the post-menopausal women receiving too little chemotherapy.

Question What are the potential hazards of cytotoxic therapy.

Answer

1 Marrow depression.
2 Alopecia.
3 Severe nausea and vomiting.
4 Psychiatric morbidity.
5 Amenorrhoea in the pre-menopausal woman.

Comment In one British trial 29 per cent of patients volunteered that they would never repeat their treatment and in an American trial 30 per cent of women could not continue.

Question What is meant by the term 'disease-free interval'.

Answer This is the term applied to that interval of time between the initial treatment of the tumour and its recurrence. There is, however, no strong evidence as yet that prolongation of the disease free interval necessarily prolongs survival. However, if all the various trials of cytotoxic agents are summated there is a suggestion that in node positive patients overall survival is prolonged.

Comment Two years later the patient complained of a thickening in the axilla and in view of her natural fear the axilla was re-explored. However, no malignant tissue was found but one year later she developed a nodule in the medial end of her mastectomy scar. This was excised with an adequate ellipse of skin and the nodule was found to be malignant. One year later further nodules appeared and in view of the apparent progression despite Tamoxifen her medication was changed to norethisterone acetate 10 mg tds (SH420 Schering), a progestin.

Question What are the side effects of this drug.

Answer Relatively no side effects are observed but in high doses a Cushing-like syndrome may develop associated with tremor and sweating.

Comment In many clinics this drug has been superceded by megestrol acetate (Megace, Bristol).

Question What is the mode of action of the progestins in carcinoma of the breast.

Answer No precise biological explanation is available. One suggestion

213

is that the progestins interfere with the nuclear-binding of the oestrogen receptor complex thus modifying the oestrogen-induced response in the cell.

Question What other hormonal preparations have been used in an attempt to modify tumour growth.

Answer

1   Androgens. In general these drugs are no longer used because of the highly undesirable side effect of virilization which may be accompanied by acne, hirsutism, increased libido and clitoral hypertrophy. However, these drugs may produce such a dramatic remission of bone metastases that hypercalcaemia occurs. In all reported series their effect on visceral and soft tissue metastases is much less marked.

2   Oestrogens. The use of oestrogens: 0.1 mg ethinyloestradiol tds (Lynoral, Organon) has been shown to be particularly effective in post-menopausal women. Its exact mode of action remains questionable. Several suggestions have been put forward including the hypothesis that excessive circulating oestrogens may have a direct toxic effect on the tumour cell.

The undesirable side effects of oestrogen therapy include:

(a) Nausea and even vomiting. This can be reduced by taking the drug in the middle of a meal.

(b) Fluid retention which may, of course, in the elderly woman lead to heart failure.

(c) Breakthrough or withdrawal bleeding in the post-menopausal woman.

Question Has hormone therapy ever been known to cure a patient.

Answer No.

Question Approximately what percentage of women respond to hormonal manipulation.

Answer Approximately one-third.

Question How long would you administer a hormone before declaring it valueless.

Answer Approximately three months.

Comment After four months treatment further nodules developed in the immediate vicinity of the scar.

Question What treatment can now be offered.

Answer Hormone suppression can be tried. This method of treatment is based on the work of Charles Huggins of Chicago who was primarily interested in the effects of castration on carcinoma of the prostate. However, presumably after reading the original paper by Beatson he extended his work to encompass carcinoma of the breast in women. This led to the introduction first of oophorectomy and later, following the discovery and manufacture of corticosteroids, of adrenalectomy and later hypophysectomy.

It has been shown that in approximately one-third of pre-menopausal patients with advanced disease surgical castration produces a temporary remission but that in the post-menopausal female, defined as a woman two years after the last missed period little benefit accrues from this manoeuvre. So far as adrenalectomy is concerned this operation is again attended by about a 30 per cent remission rate.

Question What is the best clinical indicator of a possible response to adrenalectomy.

Answer A previous response to oophorectomy.

Question What laboratory test indicates a probable response.

Answer A high level of oestrogen receptors in the tumour.

Question What is the mode of action of adrenalectomy.

Answer The adrenal cortex produces no oestrogens but secretes androstenedione which is converted into oestrogen in peripheral tissue and in the post-menopausal woman this pathway is responsible for nearly all the circulating oestrogen.

Question What treatment has now superceded surgical adrenalectomy.

Answer Treatment with the drug aminoglutethimide (Orimeten, Ciba).

Question What is the mechanism of action of this drug.

Answer This drug blocks the conversion of cholesterol to pregnenolone, reduces the production of all steroids from the adrenal cortex and also inhibits the aromatization of androstendione to oestrogens in the peripheral tissues. It has been shown, that by this dual action, it reduces the level of circulating oestradiol to that found after surgical adrenalectomy in the post-menopausal woman. This drug does not, however, affect the secretion of androgens. However, the loss of glucocorticoid excretion necessitates some form of replacement therapy, either dexamethasone (Decadron, Merck, Sharp and Dohme) or hydrocortisone.

Question What is the normal dose schedule.

Answer

1   Aminogluthemide, 250 mg twice daily for two weeks followed by 250 mg four times a day thereafter.

2   Hydrocortisone, 100 mg daily in divided doses for two weeks followed by 40 mg daily thereafter, normally administered as 20 mg at night and 10 mg in the morning and evening.

Question What investigation should be performed at the end of 14 days.

Answer Plasma electrolyte levels. If these are reduced, i.e. if hyponatraemia is present 9-α-fluorohydrocortisone, 0.1 mg daily should be given.

Question What adverse effects have been reported following the administration of aminogluthemide.

Answer Skin rashes, lethargy (approximately 40 per cent), ataxia, nystagmus, confusion (approximately 10 per cent), gastrointestinal disturbance, hypothyroidism and virilism. However, apart from hypothyroidism and virilism the effects are usually transient and in only some 10 per cent of patients has the administration of this drug had to be stopped.

Question Why should hypothyroidism occur.

Answer Because aminogluthemide can suppress thyroxine production.

Question Why should virilism occur.

Answer Because androgen secretion is not suppressed.

Comment In this patient no significant side-effects occurred and the local disease was stabilized for approximately one year, the skin nodules entirely disappearing. Thereafter the local condition again degenerated and multiple new skin nodules developed.

Question Hormonal manipulation having failed, what can this patient be offered.

Answer Cytotoxic therapy. Both single and multiple agent therapy have been advocated by numerous authors. The results reported show wide variation, e.g. using cyclophosphamide, response rates varying between 10 and 62 per cent have been reported whereas using multiple agent therapy the response rates vary between 50 and 90 per cent.

One common drug combination in use is as follows:
Day 1: oral cyclophosphamide, 50 mg twice daily. 500 mg 5-fluorouracil, 25 mg methotrexate, 5 mg vinblastine are sequentially administered via an intravenous infusion of 300 ml of sodium chloride.
Day 8: repeat infusion.
Day 15: Cease cyclophosphamide and repeat infusion.
Four weeks later recommence the cycle if the white blood count has remained above 3000×10^9/l.

Comment This patient was so upset by the first course of cytotoxic therapy that she refused to contemplate any further treatment.

Question What can now be done.

Answer Local excision of the area leaving the wound open and using a foam elastomer stent as a dressing once granulation tissue has formed on the raw surface.

Comment This treatment, i.e. wide local excision, was performed on several occasions and it was not until two years later that visceral (hepatic) metastases developed and at the same time the patient became exceedingly breathless. Physical examination revealed no apparent changes in the lung fields but several ominous physical signs were found:

(a) the external jugular veins were distended.

(b) percussion revealed apparent cardiac enlargement.

(c) the blood pressure was low compared to previous measurements.

(d) the pulse volume was small.

Question What do these physical signs suggest.

Answer A malignant pericardial effusion associated with cardiac tamponade.

Question What are the radiological features of this condition.

Answer Generalized enlargement of the cardiac shadow, the heart shadow enlarging both to the left and to the right. Both lateral borders become smoothly convex (Fig. 21.1).

Question What are the commoner causes of breathlessness in a patient suffering from carcinoma of the breast.

Answer

1   A malignant pleural effusion.

2   Lymphangitis carcinomatosis of the lungs.

Question What is the treatment of a pericardial effusion.

Answer Aspiration of the pericardial sac.

Comment Despite two taps and the instillation of bleomycin into the pericardium this patient's condition deteriorated rapidly and she died. This patient survived for some 17 years following the diagnosis of cancer of the breast and manifested generalized disease only in the last few months of life. Since subclinical cancer of the breast may be present for approximately 10 years prior to the clinical diagnosis this patient must have had considerable natural immunity to the disease. Her longevity was not initially, at least, due to a slow growth rate since the skin nodules increased in number and size at an alarming rate, neither can it have been due to hormonal control since both additive and subtraction therapy appeared to cause little change in her visible disease although medical adrenalectomy produced a recession lasting approximately one year.

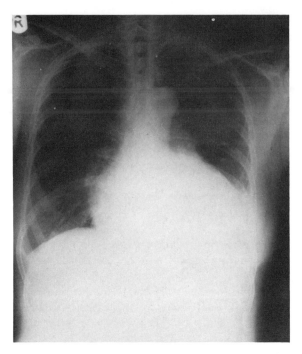

21.1

Question At no time did this patient complain of bone pain. Would you consider this unusual.

Answer Yes. Carcinoma of the breast commonly disseminates to the skeleton, particularly to the spine, ribs and pelvis although any bone may become involved.

Question What investigations are of value in establishing the presence of osseous metastases.

Answer

1 Plain X-rays of the skeleton. This investigation is of limited value since 40 per cent of the calcium content of the bone must disappear before an osteolytic metastasis is plainly visible. It has also been shown that the smallest detectable lesion is between 1–1.5 cm. The earliest radiological evidence of an osseous metastasis is an alteration in the trabecular structure of this medullary bone so that the pattern of the lamellar first becomes irregular and is later lost. Osteolytic and osteoplastic lesions occur in about 35 per cent of affected patients and osteoplastic lesion in 10 per cent.

2 Skeletal scintiscan. This is performed following the injection of 10–15 mCi of 99^mTc-hydroxyethylidine disodium phosphate, a bone

seeking nuclide. It is taken up in areas in which new bone is being laid down in an attempt to repair the destruction caused by tumour. When new bone is being formed a zone of increased uptake occurs, the 'hot spot'. It is estimated that a bone scan shows an abnormality several months before conventional X-rays become positive. However, note should be taken that benign bone disease such as the arthritides will all produce significant abnormalities.

3   When widespread osseous metastases are present the urinary calcium excretion, alkaline phosphatase and plasma phosphate may all be abnormally elevated and in addition the urinary hydroxyproline level may rise due to the degradation of bone collagen.

Question What treatment can alleviate the pain associated with bone metastases.

Answer

1   Hormonal therapy may lead to rapid alleviation of pain.

2   Relatively small doses of radiotherapy, 12 Gy, may also produce good palliation.

Comment This patient survived for some 17 years following the initial diagnosis of a Stage I cancer of the breast manifesting generalized disease only in the last few weeks of life. She illustrates the variable course this disease may take and the individuality of response. Throughout the entire period she was kept fully informed of each development and its significance.

22

A Caucasian female 18 years of age presented complaining of a gradually increasing mass in the right side of the neck, first noted two years prior to admission. Two weeks previously she had noted pain in the swelling when swallowing. In addition she also complained of the following:

1 Irritability.
2 Palpitations.
3 Increasing thirst.
4 Increased perspiration.
5 Weight gain of 7 kilograms in six months.

Previous medical history No significant ill health apart from an attack of glandular fever 10 years previously

Physical examination Inspection revealed an obvious goitre restricted to the right side of the neck. There were no obvious signs of thyrotoxicosis (see Viva 27). Palpation revealed a smooth, soft swelling in the right lobe of the thyroid. The swelling moved freely on swallowing.

Cardiovascular system	No abnormality detected.
Respiratory system	No abnormality detected.
Central nervous system	No abnormality detected. In particular there was no evidence of a tremor, no evidence of muscular weakness and no evidence of excessive perspiration.

Question What are the possible causes of a solitary swelling of the thyroid in a girl of 18 years.

Answer

1 The most probable cause of a solitary swelling with the physical signs already described in a girl of this age is a differentiated carcinoma of the thyroid.

2 A solitary cyst.

3 In view of her symptoms a solitary toxic thyroid nodule. These, however, are seldom larger than 3 cm in diameter.

Question What investigations are required.

Answer

1 In view of the symptoms suggestive of thyrotoxicosis the thyroid hormone levels should be established. These proved to be normal.

2 Ultrasound examination of the swelling. This will differentiate a solid from a cystic swelling.

In this patient the mass in the neck proved, on ultrasonography, to be solid.

Question Is thyroid scanning of great value.

Answer No, although should the nodule prove to be 'cold', i.e. not taking up I^{131}, it favours a diagnosis of malignancy. However, a small proportion of well differentiated thyroid tumours take up iodine equally as well as the surrounding normal tissues.

Comment The thyroid scan in this girl is shown in Fig. 22.1, which shows a 'cold' nodule.

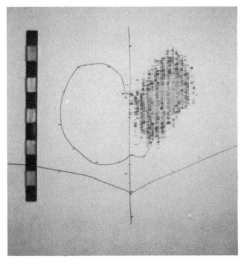

22.1

Question How common is malignant disease of the thyroid.

Answer Rare. Incidences of between 15–37 per 1 million of the population have been reported.

Question Classify the histological types of malignant disease occurring in the thyroid and indicate their appropriate frequency.

Answer The types of malignancy occurring in the thyroid can be divided into four major groups.

1 Anaplastic.
2 Differentiated.
3 Medullary.
4 Lymphosarcoma.

Approximately 40 per cent of all tumours are anaplastic but the incidence of the different types of differentiated tumours differs in the various series examined.

One large recently reported series from the Houston Tumour centre found the following incidence of the various types of differentiated tumour:

1　Mixed papillary and follicular, 65 per cent.
2　Papillary, 14.8 per cent.
3　Follicular, 15.3 per cent.
4　Hurtle cell tumours, 4.9 per cent.

Question Describe the chief macroscopic features of the common thyroid tumours.

Answer

1　Anaplastic: these tumours are unencapsulated extending widely throughout the gland and so distorting its shape. Involvement of extrathyroidal structures has frequently taken place at the time of clinical diagnosis. Their consistency varies; they may be stony-hard throughout or hard in some places and soft and friable in others.

2　Papillary: these tumours are usually unencapsulated and may be multiple. Several discrete nodules, frequently several centimetres in diameter, are present. In 40 per cent of specimens multiple foci are present in the same lobe and in 20 per cent nodules are also found in the contralateral lobe. This multiplicity of lesions is believed to be due to intrathyroidal lymphatic spread. There is a tendency for cystic degeneration to occur in both the primary tumour and its metastases, the latter developing principally in the cervical lymph nodes.

3　Follicular: this is the only tumour of the thyroid which appears to be encapsulated although invasion and penetration of the capsule can sometimes be seen with the naked eye.

Question Describe the histological pattern of pure papillary and follicular tumours.

Answer Papillary tumours are composed of columnar epithelium which is thrown into folds which form papillary projections within which are connective tissue stalks. Concentrically layered deposits of calcium, the psammoma bodies are commonly found.

Follicular tumours, in contrast, are composed of follicles of varying sizes intermixed with solid sheets of cells which may exhibit a varying degree of mitosis.

Whereas papillary tumours metastasize to the adjacent pretracheal and deep cervical lymph nodes, tumours of follicular type frequently invade the adjacent thyroid parenchyma and the blood vessels giving rise to distant metasases.

Question What is the biological behaviour of mixed well-differentiated tumours.

Answer Their behaviour appears to follow that of the major histological component. Thus a papillary tumour containing follicular elements metastases to adjacent lymph nodes whereas a follicular carcinoma containing papillary elements metastases via the blood stream.

Question What is the chief factor which determines the prognosis in follicular carcinoma.

Answer The age of the patient. In young patients malignant follicular tumours appear to be slow growing and even when the cervical nodes are involved only a small percentage of sufferers die as a direct result of tumour growth whereas in the older patient over 40 years of age such tumours appear to be more aggressive, are frequently extrathyroidal and a relatively high proportion, 15–20 per cent, of patients die as a direct consequence of tumour growth.

Question What factor chiefly determines the prognosis in papillary cancer.

Answer The invasiveness of the tumour. With minimal invasion of the capsule the prognosis is excellent but breaching of the capsule leads to death within five years in approximately 50 per cent of sufferers.

Question Place well differentiated thyroid tumours in order of aggressiveness.

Answer Papillary, mixed, follicular and Hürthe cell.

Question Since the evidence in this patient suggests the presence of a malignant thyroid lesion, should a needle biopsy be performed.

Answer The diagnostic accuracy of needle biopsy depends upon the clinic in which it is performed. A study of the literature suggests that a high degree of accuracy can be achieved in clinics in which the technique is frequently and constantly in use. Where it is seldom used it appears to be of little value. It is particularly difficult even for an experienced histopathologist to distinguish a benign from a malignant follicular lesion unless he is able to examine the capsule for evidence of invasion.

Should, ultrasound indicate that a mass in the thyroid is wholly cystic however, aspiration should be attempted.

Comment In this patient an 'open' biopsy was performed. Through an adequate neck incision the thyroid was explored. Both lobes were exposed. A mass some 70×55 mm in size was found in the right lobe whereas the left lobe appeared to be normal both on inspection and to palpation. A right haemithyroidectomy was, therefore, performed and the left lobe left *in situ*. The neck wound was then closed without drainage. The gland was sectioned and an encapsulated mass composed of whitish variegated tissue found. Histology later

223

confirmed that this tumour was a mixed follicular and papillary carcinoma with invasion, but not penetration, of the connective tissue capsule.

Comment In this patient no further action was taken.

Question What comment would you make on this decision.

Answer Many surgeons would consider that the treatment has been inadequate. They would argue that by leaving the left lobe *in situ* there is a risk of recurrence within the thyroid itself. This opinion is based on the fact that involvement of the contralateral lobe is present in 20 per cent of patients at the time of the initial operation. However, in a patient of this age, had the tumour been predominantly papillary in type many surgeons would leave the residual thyroid tissue *in situ* recognizing that such tumours in young patients run a particularly benign course even when cervical lymph node metastases are present.

In predominantly follicular tumours a second argument advanced in favour of total thyroidectomy is the impossibility of detecting and treating systemic metastases by radioactive iodine if normal thyroid tissue is left *in situ* since I^{131} will be preferentially taken up by the normal tissue.

Question Having regard to previous comments, if metastases developed in this patient where would you expect them.

Answer Bone, breast or lungs.

Question Do systemic metastases take up radioactive iodine as well as the primary tumour.

Answer Very rarely even when they are fully differentiated.

Question What are the commonest manifestions of osseous metastases.

Answer

1 Bone pain.
2 Pathological fracture.
3 A palpable tumour if the affected bone is superficial, e.g. the lower end of the radius.

Question What are the commonest manifestions of pulmonary metastases.

Answer

1 Pleuritic pain.
2 Breathlessness due to the development of a pleural effusion.
3 Haemoptyses.

Question What is meant by the term total thyroidectomy.

Answer The literature on thyroid surgery is slightly confusing. Some surgeons would argue that a total thyroidectomy is the removal of all thyroid tissue whereas others interpret the term to mean the total removal of one lobe and the removal of the greater part of the contralateral lobe leaving only a sliver of the gland in order to prevent damage to the recurrent laryngeal nerve and parathyroid glands.

Question If a total thyroidectomy is performed, how do you preserve parathyroid function.

Answer Carefully isolate one or more parathyroid glands on the side opposite to the tumour and transplant them into the muscle mass of the forearm.

Question How else, other than by surgery, can the residual thyroid tissue be ablated.

Answer By following an incomplete operation with I^{131}, a dose of 50–100 mCi is normally sufficient to ablate all normal thyroid tissue.

Question What ancillary treatment is normally prescribed in patients suffering from papillary carcinoma of the thyroid.

Answer The administration of tri-iodothyronine 20 µg tds. The dose given is designed to suppress TSH secretion by the pituitary in the belief that TSH stimulates the growth of well differentiated tumours.

Comment In this patient tri-iodothyronine was commenced immediately after her recovery and she was seen at regular intervals for a period of 12 years, during which time she married and had two normal babies. The drug was stopped immediately it was known she was pregnant. However, 12 years and four months following surgery she presented with a solitary swelling approximately 2 cm in diameter on the right jugulodigastric region.

Question What would you consider to be the most probable diagnosis.

Answer It is unlikely to be anything other than a lymph node metastases arising from the thyroid.

Question What would be the correct treatment.

Answer A limited lymphatic resection.

Comment An oblique cervical incision was made and a very vascular tumour was removed from the area described. Histology of the specimen showed it to consist of a solitary lymph node invaded by a well differentiated follicular carcinoma of the thyroid.

Question Does this histological report surprise you.

Answer Yes because we have already stated that predominantly follicular carcinoma of the thyroid disseminates via the blood stream rather than by the lymphatics.

Question In view of this report should a formal block dissection of the neck be undertaken.

Answer A search of the surgical literature suggests that further surgical treatment at this time would result in little, if any, benefit to the patient.

Comment This patient has now been followed for a further three years with no further development taking place. This merely shows the complete unpredictability in the behaviour of well differentiated thyroid malignancy.

Contrast the behaviour of this type of tumour with that of anaplastic carcinoma which is nearly always inoperable at the time the diagnosis is made and which is almost universally fatal within months of the initial diagnosis.

Question What is the place of radioactive iodine in thyroid cancer.
Answer

1   Radioactive iodine can be used to ablate residual thyroid tissue thus permitting the detection of metastatic deposits, if these are functionally capable of taking up iodine.

2   It can be used to treat systemic metastases although it would appear from the literature that even well differentiated metastases take up radioactive iodine very poorly when compared to normal tissue. Furthermore, undifferentiated thyroid tissue does not take up iodine at all.

Comment In a recent retrospective survey by the Houston Tumour Clinic the results of treating 706 patients, 514 females and 192 males, suffering from differentiated tumours of the thyroid were reported. Their conclusions were as follows:

1   Patients diagnosed before the age of 40 live significantly longer than patients over 40.

2   Females suffering from well differentiated thyroid cancer live longer than males.

3   Total thyroidectomy results in a longer disease free interval and fewer recurrences.

4   Patients receiving ablative I_2 therapy have a lower frequency of recurrence but the disease free interval and survival are not significantly different.

5   That involvement of the local lymph nodes does not affect the frequency of recurrence or survival.

6   That if recurrence should occur, 50 per cent arise in the first five years and 66 per cent within 10 years.

7   That the biological behaviour of thyroid cancer is unpredictable.

23

A Caucasian female aged 55 was admitted complaining of severe right upper quadrant pain. This had begun three days prior to admission whilst the patient was driving her car. The pain, constant since its onset, had begun in the loin before radiating to the right subcostal region. She had vomited intermittently since the onset of the pain and had been constipated. She denied any urinary symptoms.

Physical medical history Six months prior to admission she had suffered a similar attack of pain associated with some vomiting which had resolved spontaneously after 48 hours.

Physical examination Inspection revealed no abnormality.

Cardiovascular system	No abnormality. Blood pressure 130/80 mmHG. Pulse rate negative.
Respiratory system	No abnormality.
Temperature	38°C.
Abdominal examination	Palpation revealed marked tenderness in the right hypochondrium together with a positive Murphy's sign.

Question What would be a working diagnosis.

Answer Biliary colic associated with acute cholecystitis.

Question What investigations would you order.

Answer

1 Plain abdominal X-ray.
2 Ultrasound of the gall bladder.
3 Full blood count.

Comment

1 Plain abdominal X-ray revealed an ill-defined enlargement of the right kidney together with a few scattered fluid levels.
2 Ultrasound revealed a large right sided solid renal mass.
3 The full blood count revealed an increase in the total nucleated cell count and an absolute increase in the number of circulating polymorphonuclear leucocytes.

Question On this evidence and in view of the history would it be reasonable to alter the clinical diagnosis or conclude that the renal tumour was an incidental finding.

Answer It would be reasonable to assume that the diagnosis of hypernephroma complicated by the development of necrosis or bleeding within the tumour was the corrected diagnosis.

Question What is the classic triad of symptoms caused by a hypernephroma.

Answer Haematuria occurs in approximately two-thirds of all patients. Loin pain occurs in approximately one-half. A palpable mass is present in approximately one-third.

According to Riches (1963) in only about 10 per cent of patients are all three symptoms present together.

Question What complication other than haemorrhage or necrosis within the tumour can cause pain in patients suffering from a hypernephroma.

Answer When bleeding occurs into the renal pelvis, clot colic may develop, a condition easily recognizable if small worm-like clots are passed *per urethram*.

Question Is the presence of a raised temperature common in patients suffering from a hypernephroma.

Answer Comparatively common, indeed an occult hypernephroma confined to the kidney is one of the rare causes of 'pyrexia of unknown origin'. The writer has performed a nephrectomy in a patient suffering from a PUO whose temperature fell to normal 48 hours after operation and remained normal over a follow up period extending for five years.

Question What rare endocrine disturbances are sometimes associated with a hypernephroma.

Answer

1 Erythrocytosis due to the production of erythropoietin.

2 Hypercalcaemia associated with hypoplastic parathyroid glands. Other even rarer endocrine manifestations are occasionally encountered caused by the production of excessive accounts of corticotrophin, gonadotrophins or prostaglandins.

Question Can the metastases from a hypernephroma cause the presenting symptom.

Answer Yes. Metastases from a hypernephroma develop most frequently in the skeleton, producing pathological fractures in affected bones and in the lungs, remaining silent or causing repeated haemoptyses or a pleural effusion.

Question What anatomical abnormality is a rare form of presentation.

Answer Extension of a left sided tumour into the left renal vein may occlude the left testicular vein causing the rapid development of a varicocele.

Question What other investigations may assist in the diagnosis of a hypernephroma prior to operation.

Answer A variety of investigations may be pursued but since ultrasonography proves that a renal mass is solid and not cystic none are required to support the diagnosis. Prior to the development of ultrasonography the normal pattern of investigation when faced with a renal mass was:

1 Intravenous pyelography (Fig. 23.1). This proves that the mass is in the kidney, the classic radiological sign being the finding of 'spider' calyces due to stretching of the calyceal system over the developing tumour. However, a similar appearance is also produced by a simple renal cyst.

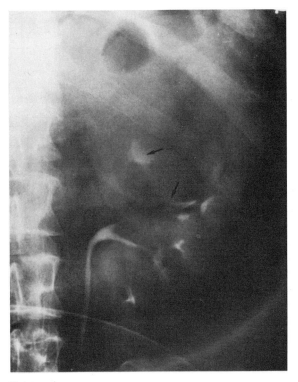

23.1

2 Aortography with selective cannulation of the appropriate renal artery. This investigation distinguishes a renal cyst from a renal tumour.

Question What are the common aortographic radiological features associated with a hypernephroma.

Answer

1 Distortion of the pattern of the major branches of the renal artery.

2 Irregular and distorted abnormal vessels.

3 Multiple arteriovenous fistulae in the substance of the kidney giving rise to early filling of the veins draining the kidney.

4 In the nephrogram stage the renal parenchyma has an irregular mottled appearance frequently referred to as 'pooling' or 'puddling' which is due to the presence of abnormal vessels within the substance of the tumour.

Question What additional investigations would be necessary to 'stage' the tumour prior to surgery.

Answer

   1 Computerized axial tomography, enhancing the renal image by means of intravenous contrast medium.

   2 Venography.

   3 Chest X-ray.

   4 Skeletal isotope survey.

Question Is the TNM classification applied to renal tumours.

Answer Yes. However, the staging of the primary tumour itself requires some modification due to the development of newer imaging techniques.

Comment In this patient the chest X-ray, arteriogram and tomography are shown in Figs 23.2, 23.3, 23.4 and 23.5.

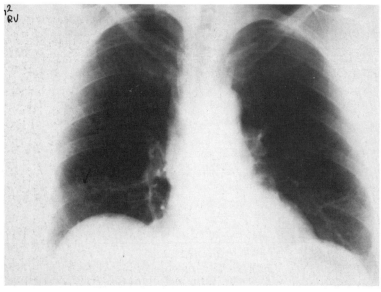

23.2

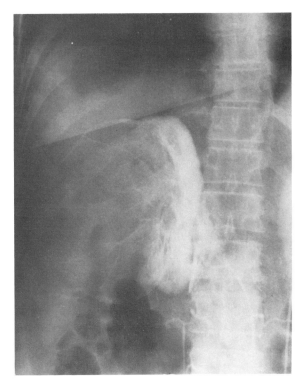

23.3

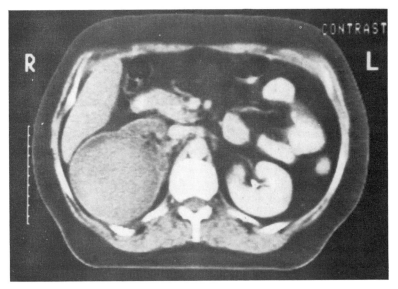

23.4

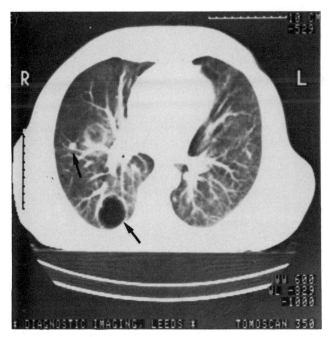

23.5

Question What do these figures show.
Answer Figure 23.2 shows the presence of a rounded opacity in the right
base, (?) a metastasis.

Figure 23.3. Selective angiogram of the right renal artery showing
the normal renal tissue compressed by a large mass lying in a lateral
position.

Figure 23.4 shows a large solid mass in the right kidney. The
kidney itself is a compressed cresentic mass lying anterior to the
bulky tumour. Further 'cuts' showed the renal vein to be incorporated
in the tumour and an absence of metases in the liver.

Figure 23.5 shows an appropriate 'cut' through the thorax in which
the rather vague mass seen in the chest X-ray is shown as a cir-
cumscribed solid mass. In addition in the posterior position a large
pulmonary 'cyst' can be seen.

Comment In this particular patient the renal tumour was embolized, the
surgeon to whose care she was transferred believing that this
technique was of value. This is a matter of debate. The generally
accepted view is that this technique may be useful for debulking, by

232

producing necrosis, massive renal tumours but that it is of little value in the average patient.

Question What materials have been used to embolize the kidney.

Answer Sterispon (Gel, Foam), Dura mater, steel coils and thrombin. This technique was originally described by Almgard in 1973. He claimed that embolization:

1 Reduces tumour bulk and hence facilitates nephrectomy.
2 Reduces blood flow making operation easier.
3 In inoperable tumours reduces haematuria.

In order to produce an infarct greater than 50 per cent of the tumour mass complete occlusion is required.

Question What operation is now performed for unilateral hypernephroma.

Answer Radical nephrectomy.

Question What does this entail.

Answer The kidney is usually approached via an anterior or thoraco-abdominal incision. The first aim is to ligate the renal artery of the affected kidney so that the extensive network of veins in the perinephric fat bleed less profusely when they are torn during mobilization of the kidney. The renal vein is then controlled in the hope that blood stream metastases will be avoided. Once the major blood vessels are controlled the upper ureter is identified and divided after which the kidney, together with the adrenal gland, the perinephric fat and Gerota's fascia is removed.

Question Assuming the tumour is confined to the kidney at the time of operation what is the prognosis.

Answer Approximately 60 per cent of patients will be alive in five years.

Question What is the gross appearance of a renal adenocarcinoma.

Answer On cross-section the tumour may be lobulated and surrounded by a pseudocapsule. The cut surface is yellow except in areas in which haemorrhage or necrosis have occurred.

Question What is the microscopic appearance.

Answer The cells of a renal adenocarcinoma are polygonal or oval and are typically arranged in a solid trabecular fashion. They possess either a clear cytoplasm which contains glycogen or a granular cytoplasm which contains large numbers of mitochondria.

Question Can distant blood-bourne metastases develop prior to the involvement of the paraortic lymph nodes.

Answer Yes. This is the argument employed against the extension of radical nephrectomy to include abdominal lymphadenectomy. Not only may blood-bourne metastases be present at the time of operation but as with the majority of cancers lymphatic spread does not necessarily occur in a uniform manner, e.g. contralateral nodes may be involved prior to apparent involvement of the ipsilateral nodes.

Question What is the incidence of bilateral hypernephroma.

Answer Bilateral tumours occur synchronously or asynchronously in three per cent of cases.

Question What treatment would be possible in cases of bilateral tumours.

Answer Assuming both tumours are operable a bilateral partial nephrectomy may be possible. Some authorities would advise bilateral nephrectomy and then after a disease free period during which the patient is maintained on dialysis a renal transplant.

Question Does spontaneous regression of renal carcinoma occur.

Answer Yes. Spontaneous regression has been reported to occur in the following tumours: hypernephroma, malignant melanoma and carcinoma of the breast. So far as melanoma is concerned spontaneous regression is nearly always associated with pregnancy and breast tumours may regress during the menopause.

Question Is pre- or post-operative adjuvant radiotherapy effective in the treatment of hypernephroma.

Answer No. The Rotterdam trial, reported in 1973, in which patients in whom no distant metastases had been demonstrated, were treated by pre-operative deep X-ray therapy showed no evidence of increased survival over matched controls. Similarly the British trial also published in 1973 drew attention to three factors which adversely affect radiotherapy.

1 Relative radioresistance.

2 Areas of necrosis and hypoxia within the tumour.

3 A dose sufficient to affect the tumour will injure surrounding normal tissues.

Question Has radiotherapy any place in the treatment of patients suffering from a hypernephroma.

Answer Yes. It can be used to treat painful osseous metastases.

Question What is the place of chemotherapy.

Answer Neither single or multiple drug regimes appear to be useful in this disease.

Question Is hormonal manipulation useful.

Answer Very little. The hormones which may occasionally influence the progression of the disease include medroxyprogesterone and testosterone propionate.

Comment This patient made an uninterrupted recovery following radical nephrectomy when she was readmitted some six months later complaining as she put it, 'of the same pain as before'. She was under investigation when she suddenly collapsed and died. Autopsy showed that she had a large posterior duodenal ulcer approximately 1.5 cm in diameter which had eroded the head of the pancreas thus causing her initial symptom of back pain. As a terminal event both severe haemorrhage and perforation had occurred into the lesser sac. An example of tunnel vision perhaps!

24

A male 61 years of age was admitted complaining of intermittent painless haematuria of several weeks duration.

Previous medical history Ten years prior to admission the patient had suffered from 'piles'. He had been treated by haemorrhoidectomy and developed anal stenosis as a result. Six years prior to admission he had developed hypertension for which he had been treated with a large variety of drugs.

Physical examination This revealed no abnormality. Rectal examination revealed a tight anal stricture.

Question What does this history suggest.

Answer The presence of a urethelial tumour in the upper or lower urinary tract.

Question What types of renal tumour occur in the adult.

Answer

    1   Clear cell carcinoma formerly known as the Gravitz tumour or hypernephroma (see Viva 23).

    2   Transitional cell tumours of the pelvis or calyces.

Question What symptoms other than bleeding may be associated with renal carcinoma.

Answer Clot colic, pyrexia, anaemia and amyloidosis. Occasionally ectopic hormone production occurs, the commonest of which is the production of erythropoietin causing cryothrocytosis.

Question What type of renal tumour occurs in childhood.

Answer Nephroblastoma (Wilm's tumour). This tumour is composed of spindle-celled tissue in which acini and tubular structures may be seen together with occasional striped muscle fibres.

Question What is the common presenting symptom of a nephroblastoma.

Answer The accidental finding of a mass in the loin. In one patient treated by the author the mother had noted the presence of the abdominal mass when dressing her five year old daughter in her kilt; the straps would not fasten.

Question What is the first investigation you would order in this patient.

Answer A midstream specimen of urine which should be examined for the presence of malignant cells and evidence of infection.

Comment In this patient both malignant transitional cells and pus cells were found in the urine.

Question What cells, if any, are found in normal urine.

Answer The most common cells found in normal urine are those derived from the superficial layers of the bladder epithelium. These are flat, oval or irregularly shaped cells varying between 20–25 μm along their largest diameter. Smaller cells, 12–15 μm in diameter originating from the deeper layers of the vesical mucosa are rarely found in normal urine but become numerous if the bladder is inflamed when in addition polymorphonuclear leucocytes, lymphocytes and histiocytes will also be present.

Question What are the characteristic features of malignant urothelial cells.

Answer

1   Single cancer cells may be seen due to lack of adhesiveness of malignant cells.

2   The nuclei are enlarged, irregular in outline, hyperchromatic and show a coarse distribution of chromatin granules.

3   Nuclear size is extremely variable.

The accuracy of exfoliative cytology is increased if separate specimens are examined on three consecutive days when positive diagnosis of between 60 and 89 per cent can be achieved.

In order to diminish the time taken and the expense of another technique which has been described is to divide one centrifuged specimen into three parts and stain each with a different stain, those recommended being Giemsa, Papanicolaou and Al Red O. Whilst Giemsa appears superior to the last two, when all three are used the accuracy of diagnosis in one reported series reached 80 per cent

Question What further investigations are required in order to assess the management of this patient.

Answer

1   An intravenous pyelogram.

2   Cystoscopy followed by multiple biopsies or complete resection of the bladder tumour, if present or possible, and a bimanual examination after complete emptying of the bladder at the termination of resection.

Question The intravenous pyelogram is shown in Figs 24.1 and 24.2. What are the chief findings.

Answer Both kidneys are secreting the contrast normally and there is no significant abnormality of the upper urinary tract. The ureters do not appear to be obstructed. The left side of the bladder is very irregular, consistent with the presence of an infiltrating carcinoma.

Comment Bimanual examination after completely emptying the bladder following resection of all visible tumour revealed a residual mobile mass involving the left wall of the bladder. Histopathological examination of the resected tumour showed that it was composed of both

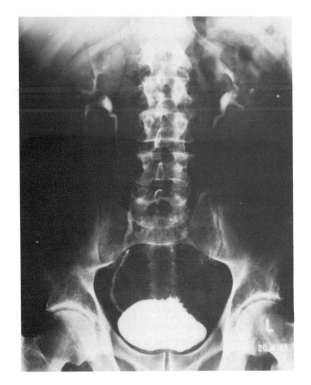

24.1

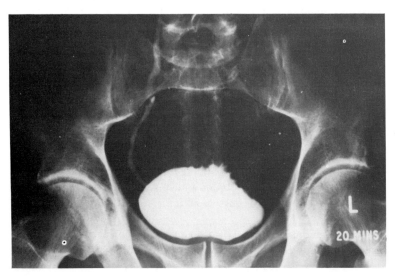

24.2

238

papillary and solid parts, the solid component invading the muscle to the limits of the resection. Areas adjacent to the tumour showed florid cystitis cystica and cystitis glandularis.

Question What is the clinical stage of this tumour.

Answer T_3 a or b.

Question What is the definition of a T_3 tumour.

Answer Stage 3 is subdivided in T_3a and T_3b.

In both, bimanual examination reveals induration or a nodular mobile mass in the bladder which persists after transurethral resection of the exophytic portion of the lesion and/or there is microscopic evidence of deep invasion of the vesical muscle.

T_3a, is a tumour invading deep into the muscle.

T_3b, is a tumour which has penetrated the vesical wall to reach the extra vesical tissues.

Question What are the definitions of a T_1 and T_2 tumour.

Answer A T_1 tumour is one that can be felt on bimanual examination prior to resection but not following resection and/or microscopically the tumour has not invaded beyond the lamina propria. This group together with papillary non-invasive carcinoma, account for approximately 80 per cent of all bladder tumours. A T_2 tumour has the same findings prior to and following resection but microscopic examination shows evidence of invasion of the superficial muscle.

Question On what evidence does the pathologist base a diagnosis of malignancy in transitional cell tumours of the bladder.

Answer In this patient the pathological diagnosis was simple since the tumour was seen invading the bladder muscle. In the absence of invasion or demonstrable metastases, however, the distinction between a simple and a malignant transitional cell tumour becomes more difficult. The WHO proposed that all urothelial tumours should be regarded as malignant whenever any deviation from the normal pattern of the vesical mucosa is found. Normally the vesical mucosa is formed of some five to seven layers of transitional cells.

Any deviation from this is indicative of anaplasia which is associated with an increase in cellularity, nuclear crowding, disturbances of cellular polarity, failure of differentiation from the base to the surface, irregularity in the size of the cells, variations in the shape of the nuclei and lastly, the presence of displaced or abnormal mitotic figures.

Question What is meant by the term papilloma of the bladder.

Answer This term is now used to describe an exophytic tumour of the bladder mucosa the fronds of which are covered by an epithelium indistinguishable from that of normal urothelium with no evidence of mitotic activity or variation in nuclear size.

Question Is the behaviour of an apparently simple papilloma entirely predictable.

Answer No. Various recorded series have demonstrated that even in patients diagnosed clinically and pathologically to be suffering from a papilloma a variable percentage eventually become invasive.

Question What is meant by the term 'carcinoma *in situ*'.

Answer This term is applied to a lesion which on endoscopic examination appears flat but in which the normal urothelium is replaced by irregular atypical cells. This type of tumour may be the forerunner of an infiltrating carcinoma.

Question How does 'carcinoma *in situ*' present.

Answer The patient may complain of dysuria rather than haematuria. Abnormal cells and pus cells may be present in the urine. Cystoscopy shows the mucosa to be roughened, thickened, irregular, indurated and haemorrhagic.

Question What growth patterns are seen in transitional cell carcinoma.

Answer

1 The exophytic or papillary.

2 The endophytic infiltrating cancer.

3 An intermediate type, the papillary infiltrating from which this particular patient was suffering.

4 Diffuse papillomatosis, this is a rare tumour. All or the greater part of the bladder wall is covered by an exophytic growth, biopsy showing either normal or anaplastic cells.

Question What other pathological types of bladder tumour occur.

Answer Squamous cell tumours. This type of tumour occurs in patients suffering from ectopia vesicae, those infested with *Schistosoma haematobium* and patients in whom squamous metaplasia has been induced by the presence of a vesical calculus. Rarely the bladder can be the site of a phaeochromocytoma or adenocarcinoma, the latter tumour being most frequently of urachal origin.

Question What chemical carcinogens cause transitional cell tumours of the bladder.

Answer α and β napthyalamine, benzidine, dichlorbenzidine and a variety of other compounds.

Question In what occupations were these chemicals used.

Answer Particularly in the chemical industry, rubber industry and by electric cable markers.

Question What is the latent period between exposure to a chemical carcinogen and the development of bladder cancer.

Answer Very long, the estimated time varying between 20 and 40 years.

Question What known bladder carcinogens are now prohibited.

Answer 2-naphthylamine, benzidine, 4-aminobiphenyl and 4-nitro-biphenyl and their salts. In addition there is a comprehensive list of controlled substances in which great care is taken to make sure that workers do not come into direct contact with the material, i.e. α-tolidine and that workers processing such chemicals have a urinary cytology performed at six monthly intervals.

Question What further investigations may indicate the choice of treatment.

Answer

1 Ultrasonography. Ultrasonography of the bladder can be used to assess the depth of infiltration of a bladder tumour. It is, therefore, particularly valuable when technical problems such as obesity make bimanual examination unsatisfactory.

2 CAT and lymphangiography. These two investigations are considered together because each may provide additional information but each has limitations. Thus CAT can be used for tumour staging when the accuracy is approximately 80 per cent.

The density difference between urine (10–20 HV) and tumour tissue (generally 30–50 HV) is usually sufficient for the identification of exophytic tumours greater than 1.5 cm in diameter. Intramural extension can also be identified but signs of local thickening of the bladder wall and irregularity of the usual homogeneously rounded configuration can be caused by oedema and fibrosis due to previous transurethral surgery or radiotherapy. In general terms the reliability of CAT increases with the progression of malignancy.

So far as the identification of lymph node metastases is concerned CAT gives a greater false positive rate than does lymphangiography whereas the latter gives a greater false negative rate because whilst bipedal lymphangiography results in the contrast medium filling the inguinal, external common iliac and para-aortic nodes the site of dissemination of bladder tumours is into the internal iliac group of nodes which are not normally visualized. A further point to recognize is that CAT identifies enlargement of the lymph nodes which may not necessarily be infiltrated with neoplastic tissue. However, in centres where CAT is available this investigation has virtually displaced lymphangiography.

3 In patients in whom simple or radical cystectomy is being considered as the treatment a bone scan should be performed to exclude the presence of bony skeletal metastases.

Question What complications may follow transurethral resection of a bladder tumour.

Answer

1 Perforation of the bladder recognized by the failure of the irrigating fluid to be returned, and later by signs of pelvic irritation.

2 Haemorrhage resulting in clot retention.

Question What information, other than the depth of infiltration, is provided by multiple biopsies.

Answer The degree of differentiation of the tumour.

Question How is this graded.

Answer

G0: No evidence of anaplasia (papilloma).

G1: Low grade malignancy (differentiation).

G2: Medium grade malignancy (differentiation).

G3: High grade malignancy (undifferentiated).

GX: Grade cannot be assessed.

Comment The histological report on the chippings removed from this patient showed that the tumour was undifferentiated (G3).

Question What are the alternative methods of treatment available for this patient.

Answer

1 Radiotherapy.

2 Radiotherapy followed by cystectomy and urinary division.

3 Cystectomy together with urinary diversion.

Comment The problem facing the surgeon dealing with such a patient is that there is no individual series of patients treated either by a single surgeon or as part of a cohort study which shows statistically significant differences in the end results.

Question What are the complications associated with radiotherapy.

Answer

1 Early: severe non specific inflammation of both the bladder and rectum leading to severe dysuria, tenesmus and diarrhoea.

2 Late:

(a) The bladder may contract producing a degree of frequency amounting to incontinence.

(b) Vesical and rectal telangiectasis may develop, the former leading to such severe bleeding that control can only be established by cystectomy.

(c) Radiation necrosis of the bowel leading to perforation and peritonitis.

Such complications occur in approximately 10 per cent of all patients treated.

Question What are the theoretical advantages of radiotherapy prior to cystectomy.

Answer The danger of spilling viable cancer cells into the pelvis is considerably reduced.

Question What is the disadvantage of pre-operative radiotherapy.

Answer The operation is made technically more difficult and in consequence is followed by a higher morbidity and mortality.

Question What types of cystectomy have been described.

Answer

1 Simple total cystectomy in which the plane of dissection is primarily extraperitoneal immediately peripheral to the vesical muscle. In the male the prostate and seminal vesicles are removed and in the female varying portions of the urethra.

2 Radical cystectomy in which the plane of dissection follows the muscular and bony walls of the pelvis rather than the bladder wall. The lymph nodes distal to the bifurcation of the common iliac artery are removed. In the male the prostate together with the seminal vesicles, and even the whole length of the urethra may be removed, and in the female the uterus and its adnexa together with the whole of the urethra and the anterior vaginal wall.

Question What are the disadvantages of cystectomy.

Answer

1 There is a considerable mortality of the order of 10 per cent. The mortality can be reduced by performing the operation in two stages, i.e. first fashioning the ileal conduit and diverting the urinary flow and then at a second stage some six weeks later performing the cystectomy. The theoretical disadvantage of the two stage procedure is the delay between the two stages gives time for a very aggressive tumour to metastasize.

2 The patient loses both normal urinary and sexual activity.

Question What are the chief causes of death following cystectomy.

Answer 50 per cent of the mortality is associated with the performance of a long operation frequently in an elderly patient. Thus the common causes of death include:

1 Myocardial infarction.

2 Cerebrovascular accidents.

3 Pulmonary complications.

The chief causes of death which are directly associated with the surgical procedure itself are the development of urinary and/or faecal fistulae due to the breakdown of the various anastomoses. Reoperation on these complications results in further mortality due to the non-specific causes listed above and also from specific causes such as peritonitis. Less commonly intestinal obstruction occurs which may also necessitate reoperation.

Common complications not necessarily resulting in death include non-fatal cardiopulmonary conditions, paralytic ileus and wound infection.

Comment In many centres the operation of radical cystectomy has been abandoned because it has been found in all the series reported that nodal involvement has a dramatic effect on survival. In some American centres if prior investigation or a trial dissection reveals that more than two nodes are involved the operation is abandoned.

Question What is the ultimate prognosis in stage T_3 bladder cancer.

Answer In the absence of nodal involvement between 33 and 50 per cent of the patients will be alive and well without signs of recurrence at five years.

Question Has chemotherapy any part to play in the treatment of advanced bladder cancer.

Answer Very little.

Comment This patient was severely hypertensive but it was decided to treat him by a two stage cystectomy. At the first stage an ileal conduit was fashioned and at that time it was noted that there was no evidence of extravesical spread.

His recovery from this operation was slightly delayed by some leakage from a uretero-ileal anastomosis which occurred on the fifth day but which settled without interference. He was discharged home on the 13th post-operative day. Six weeks later he was admitted for cystectomy which was performed using cephradine and metranidazole as prophylactic antibiotics. His post-operative course was interrupted by an intermittent pyrexia which settled spontaneously. This was considered to be due to a small pelvic collection since his total nucleated cell count rose to 19×10^9/l. He did not, however, manifest any of the usual symptoms of a pelvic abscess such as mucus diarrhoea and tenesmus but investigation revealed no alternative source for his intermittent pyrexia. He was discharged home on the 19th post-operative day.

His follow up extends for only 18 months but he remains well. The pathological report showed that the tumour had invaded the bladder wall on a wide front, only a rim 1 mm in thickness separating it from the perivesical tissues. Widespread cystitis cystica and glandularis was present surrounding the tumour. No lymph nodes were identified. Two small foci of adenocarcinoma were found in the prostate. Therefore the pathological diagnosis was Grade 3, Stage pT3, pNx.

Question What does the classification pNx mean.

Answer That since no lymph nodes have been found in the specimen the minimum requirements to assess the regional and/or juxtaregional lymph nodes have not been met.

Question What are cystitis cystica and cystitis glandularis.

Answer In cystitis cystica spaces are seen in the lamina propria lined by normal transitional epithelium and in the latter the spaces are lined by either tall columnar or pseudostratified mucous epithelium. Both these conditions are frequently seen at the advancing edges of many vesical carcinomata

Question Is the presence of two occult foci of prostatic cancer significant.

Answer No. If these foci had been discovered following a routine retropubic prostatectomy the prognosis has been found to be as good as in an age-matched control population.

25

A male aged 33 years of age attended the out-patient department complaining of swelling of his right testes which he had first observed some four weeks previously. He had initially dismissed this abnormality as of little importance since immediately prior to noting the swelling he had sustained a minor injury to his scrotum during a rugby match.

Previous medical history Nil.

Physical examination Inspection revealed nothing other than an obvious swelling in the right side of the scrotum. Palpation of the scrotum revealed a non-tender enlarged right testes approximately three times the size of the testes in the opposite side of the scrotum. The epididymis was impalpable and the cord was not thickened.

Question What are the commonest causes of a chronic painless enlargement of the body of the testes.

Answer
    1 A normal testes may appear enlarged if the opposite testes is atrophic.
    2 A haematocele. Following a scrotal injury bleeding may distend the tunica vaginalis. The blood later organizes to produce a hard insensitive mass.
    3 Gumma.
    4 True tumours of the testes.

Question What are the common causes of an acute painful enlargement of the testes.

Answer
    1 Mumps orchitis.
    2 Various causes of acute epididymo-orchitis.
    3 Granulomatous orchitis.

Question What may cause atrophy of the testes.

Answer Testicular atrophy may be unilateral or bilateral.
    Unilateral atrophy may be caused by:
    1 Mumps.
    2 Devascularization caused by:
      (a) A natural process such as unrecognized or untreated torsion of the testes.
      (b) Damage to the testicular vessels during a hernia repair.
    Bilateral atrophy follows hormonal disturbances causing hyperoestronism:

1   The administration of oestrogens for the treatment of metastatic bone lesions in carcinoma of the prostate.

2   Failure to denature natural oestrogens as in chronic liver disease.

3   Oestrogen secreting tumours such as Sertoli-cell or Leydig cell tumours of the testes.

Question What are the possible diagnoses in this patient.

Answer In view of the rugby injury the possibility of a haematocele arises but a testicular tumour is more probable.

Question What other condition may follow severe physical activity such as rugby.

Answer In a younger individual torsion may occur. This is an extremely painful condition. It may spontaneously resolve, the torsion unwinding itself or it may progress to cause gangrene of the testes. Frequently the congenital abnormality predisposing to torsion of one testes is present on the opposite side. Therefore, when operating upon the affected side the opposite testes should be fixed so as to prevent a similar catastrophe.

Question Is a history of injury to the testes common in patients suffering from a testicular tumour.

Answer Yes. In nearly a quarter of all cases there is some history of injury. This does indicate that trauma is a causative factor but it is more probable that the injury merely draws attention to an already pre-existing condition.

Question What is the incidence of testicular neoplasms.

Answer The annual incidence is of the order of 2.5–3.0 per 100000 males. Such tumours are rare before puberty.

Question Is it possible to mistake a tumour of the testes for epididymo-orchitis.

Answer Yes. A tumour of the testes may cause pain from the outset or pain may develop during the course of the disease. The commonest cause of pain is stretching of the tunica albuginea by sudden haemorrhage into the tumour.

Question What physical signs other than swelling of the body of the testes are associated with tumours of the testes.

Answer

1   The swelling is hard in the majority of cases.

2   The enlarged testes may be smooth or irregular; the irregularity, particularly if posterior, may lead to the erroneous diagnosis of epididymo-orchitis.

3   Normal testicular sensation is absent or greatly diminished in the majority.

4   The scar of a previous orchidopexy may be found in a small percentage of patients.

5   Overt metastases may be present.

6   Gynaecomastia may develop.

7   A small hydrocele may be present.

Question What is the relationship between testicular malignancy and nondescent of the testes.

Answer The chance of malignancy in an undescended testes is approximately 40 times greater than in the normal. However, when the undescended testes is brought into the scrotum prior to the age of five or six years this increase in the incidence of malignancy is abolished although after this age orchidopexy appears to confer no benefit.

Question Which tumours present the greatest difficulty in diagnosis.

Answer Those developing in the groove between the epididymus and the body of the testes when the possibility of epididymitis may lead to a mistaken diagnosis.

Question What is the nature and natural history of granulomatous orchitis.

Answer This condition normally presents as a unilateral painful swelling of the testes which subsides after a few weeks leaving an indurated organ of diminished sensitivity. The cause of the condition is unknown. The lesion is characterized by the development of an interstitial inflammatory infiltrate of lymphocytes, plasma cells and occasional eosinophils. There is atrophy of the germinal epithelium. The cellular infiltrate has led to the suggestion that the condition is of auto-immune pathogenesis. A further suggestion is that leakage of tubular contents into the interstitium following injury to the testes may provoke this reaction.

Question What is the pathological picture of a gumma of the testes.

Answer A gumma produces extensive dull yellowish necrotic areas within the body of the testes. Histologically these areas of parenchymal necrosis are surrounded by a layer of connective tissue infiltrated with lymphocytes and plasma cells. Since gummata only occur in the tertiary stage of syphilis and eventually lead to atrophy they should seldom present a diagnostic problem.

Question What simple investigation will confirm the presence of a testicular tumour.

Answer Ultrasonography. Testicular tumours may produce echo poor mass lesions or echogenic areas due to fibrosis or calcification, the latter being typical of germ cell tumours. Tumours as small as 0.5 cm, i.e. impalpable tumours may be found by this method.

Question The ultrasonic examination of the testes is shown in Figs 25.1 and 25.2 what do these show.

Answer Figure 25.1 shows the ultrasonic appearance of the normal left testes and Fig. 25.2, the ultrasonic appearance of the abnormal right

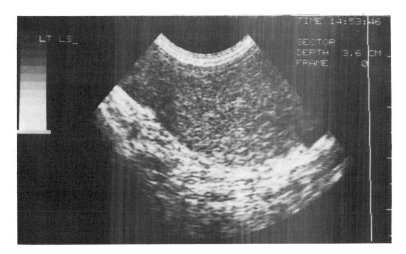

25.1

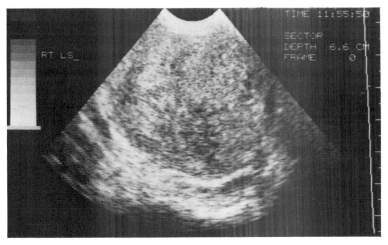

25.2

testes which is enlarged and has multiple echogenic areas suggesting the diagnosis of a teratoma.

Question What types of testicular tumour are now recognized.

Answer The situation is complicated by the variety of classifications. The major competing classifications are those of the British Testicular Tumour Panel and of the World Health Organization. Below are listed the commonest tumours.

The BTTP system is as follows:

1   Seminoma.

2 Teratoma differentiated (TD).
3 Malignant teratoma intermediate (MTI).
4 Malignant teratoma undifferentiated (MTU).
5 Malignant teratoma trophoblastic (MTT).
6 Yolk sac tumour.
7 Combined tumours in which both teratomatous and seminomatous components can be identified. The prognosis in this group is that of the teratomatous component.
8 Malignant lymphoma.

The WHO classification is as follows:

1 Seminoma.
2 Teratoma:
(a) mature.
(b) immature.
(c) with malignant transformation.
3 Embryonal carcinoma.
4 Yolk sac tumours.
5 Choriocarcinoma.
6 Tumours of more than one histological type. Embryonal carcinoma with teratoma and/or seminoma.
7 Malignant lymphoma.

In addition to the above the following tumours also occur in the testes.
1 The interstitial cell tumour (Leydig).
2 The mesenchymal tumour (Sertoli-cell tumours).

Question Which is the commonest testicular tumour.

Answer Seminoma. This tumour accounts for approximately 40 per cent of all testicular tumours. The peak incidence is in the fourth decade and two types are generally recognized, the classical and the spermatocytic, the former comprising over 90 per cent of the whole group.

Question What are the gross and microscopic appearances of a seminoma.

Answer This tumour forms a well demarcated mass which is uniform in appearance, whitish in colour with occasional yellow areas of necrosis. Microscopically the lesion is composed of fairly uniform sheets of cells, round or polygonal in shape with a finely granular cytoplasm. Multi-nucleated tumour giant cells may be present in some cases and these cells can be shown to contain human chorionic gonadotrophin (HCG). Areas of testicular scarring believed to be caused by tumour regression are sometimes seen and indeed in 1965 Azzopardi and Hoffman described a patient in whom overt metastatic disease was present in the absence of any apparently viable tumour cells in the testes.

Approximately 10 per cent of patients suffering from a seminoma have detectable metastases when first seen.

Question What is the frequency of teratoma.

Answer Teratomata comprise approximately one-third of all testicular tumours and arise from the germ cells.

Question At what age are teratoma most common.

Answer In the third decade. These tumours are rare after 50 years of age. The most primitive of these tumours is the malignant teratoma undifferentiated (MTU) which is the equivalent to an embryonal carcinoma. Such tumours are largely solid whereas the most differentiated tumours of this group, teratoma differentiated (TD), which are relatively rare, are usually cystic. Whereas the latter tumour rarely behaves in a malignant fashion in children this is not so in adults.

Question What staging system has been proposed for testicular tumours.

Answer A number of different staging systems have been described, the majority now taking into account not only the site of extratesticular spread but also the size of the metastases.

Stage I. No evidence of spread present outside the testes.

Stage II. Infradiaphragmatic nodal involvement. In general lymphatic spread first involves the lymph nodes in the region of the renal veins and then passes retrogradely to involve the iliac nodes.

Stage IIA, the maximum diameter of the involved nodes is less than 2 cm.

Stage IIB, the maximum diameter of the involved nodes is between 2 and 5 cm.

Stage IIC, the maximum diameter of the involved nodes is greater than 5 cm.

Stage III. Both infra and supradiaphragmatic nodal involvement is present.

Stage IV. Extension of the tumour to extralymphatic sites has occurred. The commonest sites for such spread being the lungs and the liver.

Question What are the essential investigations prior to proceeding to orchidectomy in suspected cases of testicular malignancy.

Answer

1 Estimation of the tumour markers alpha fetoprotein and chorionic gonadotrophin. It has now been shown that a large proportion of patients suffering from malignant teratoma have AFP, HCG or both in their blood. An elevated level of these markers is a reliable indication of the presence of active malignant teratomatous tissue, with the exception of malignant trophoblastic teratoma AFP is somewhat more specific and more frequently detected. However, other causes of a rise in AFP and HCG should be considered such as gastrointestinal malignant disease.

In malignant teratoma the range of values for AFP may vary from

251

normal to many thousand times the normal, the absolute concentration depending on the laboratory performing the assay.

HCG is a sensitive tumour marker. This glycoprotein hormone is synthesized by trophoblastic tissues. The most significant contribution to clinical medicine has been in the monitoring of gestational choriocarcinoma.

Whereas an elevated AFP is not found in pure seminomata approximately 10 per cent of these tumours are associated with a rise in the β subunit of HCG.

2   Chest radiograph.

3   Lymphangiography. Bipedal lymphangiography was introduced in the early 1960s to assess the condition of the abdominal lymph nodes. Unfortunately lymph nodes situated in the upper para-aortic region, the renal and splenic hilum, the porta hepatis and the mesentery are not opacified by lymphangiography. This is particularly well shown in Fig. 25.3 in which the iliac lymph nodes are well demonstrated but the superior nodes are not. The iliac nodes appear to be enlarged suggesting malignant involvement but the enlargement is bilateral, symmetrical and the texture of the nodes is normal, all factors negating this possibility.

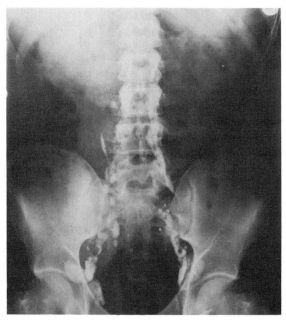

25.3

4 Ultrasonography. Any lymph node which can be detected by ultrasonography is enlarged although the cause need not necessarily be malignant involvement. However, routine ultrasonography combined with sequential estimation of AFP and HCG has proved useful in following patients suffering from testicular malignancy.

5 Computerized axial tomography, if available, can also be used to assess the presence and size of the abdominal lymph nodes.

Comment In this patient whole body scanning revealed enlargement of the upper para-aortic nodes which appeared to be approximately 3 cm in diameter.

Question What Stage is, therefore, applicable in this patient.

Answer Stage IIB, i.e. a testicular tumour associated with infradiaphragmatic lymph nodes between 2 and 5 cm in diameter.

Question What immediate treatment is required.

Answer Orchidectomy.

Question How should this be performed.

Answer Via an inguinal incision, gently dislocating the testes from the scrotum and dividing the cord at the level of the internal ring.

Question Is local extratesticular spread ever present.

Answer Very rarely indeed because the dense tunica albuginea contains the tumour even though distant lymphatic and blood stream spread is occurring.

Question Is testicular biopsy ever justified.

Answer The only possible indication would be when a testicular swelling, in which the diagnosis is uncertain occurs in a solitary testes.

Question Is a scrotal incision ever justified.

Answer No, because a residual nodule usually develops in the scrotum which may cause concern necessitating a further surgical procedure.

Comment Examination of the operative specimen in this patient showed that the tumour was a teratoma (MTI), i.e. malignant teratoma intermediate.

Question What is the histological structure of a MTI.

Answer This tumour is intermediate in structure between the differentiated and the undifferentiated, the elements composing the tumour have the histological features of malignancy but neither fully differentiated nor completely undifferentiated tissues can be found.

Question What further investigation is required.

Answer A further blood sample for estimation of AFP and β HCG should be taken approximately one week after surgery.

Comment Orchidectomy in this patient was followed by a course of radiotherapy, a midplane dose of 3500 rads being administered over three and a half weeks. The patient was then followed for a period of 18 months during which the AFP and β-HCG levels were estimated at monthly intervals. At this point an abrupt rise in the concentration of the tumour markers developed suggesting renewed activity in the metastatic disease. A further ultrasound confirmed enlargement of the para-aortic lymph nodes (Fig. 25.4).

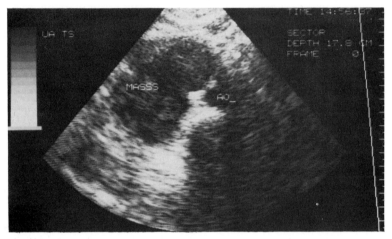

25.4

Question Is the development of recurrent para-aortic disease entirely unexpected.

Answer No. It has been repeatedly shown that cure and recurrence following orchidectomy and radiotherapy are related to the initial bulk of the abdominal node metastases. A Stage IIA tumour is followed by a low local recurrence rate and a high overall cure rate whereas when bulkier metastases are present recurrence is common and in early series only 35 per cent of such patients survived.

Question What further treatment can be given to this patient.

Answer Chemotherapy. A large number of single agents have been shown to be effective in the treatment of teratomata including mithramycin, actinomycin D, vinblastine and methotrexate. However, it is now the practise to use combinations of various drugs, e.g. cis-platinum, bleomycin and vincristine (PVB) although other drug combinations have also been described.

Question Which tumour type responds best to chemotherapy.

Answer Malignant teratoma undifferentiated (MTU) is normally followed by a better response, both temporary and permanent than malignant teratoma intermediate (MTI). Complete remission of the disease using PVB can be anticipated in about two-thirds of the patients treated.

Question What are the chief dangers associated with intensive chemotherapy.

Answer

1 Neutropenia leading to the danger of infection.
2 Thrombocytopenia leading to the possibility of haemorrhage.
3 Alopecia.
4 Stomatitis.

In addition bleomycin produces skin rashes, pigmentation and also a febrile reaction simulating influenza.

Question Does any other factor, other than histological structure, govern the response to chemotherapy.

Answer Tumour volume regardless of the agent or agents used.

Question Is chemotherapy replacing radiotherapy as first line treatment.

Answer Yes. In many centres any teratomatous tumour which has advanced beyond Stage IIA is treated by chemotherapy rather than radiotherapy. However, seminomata are extremely radiosensitive and for this tumour radiotherapy still remains the initial treatment of choice.

Question What is the place of abdominal lymphadenectomy.

Answer This technique has been used, particularly in North America, as a staging procedure in order to identify microscopic nodal involvement. In Great Britain this technique is chiefly used to debulk residual para-aortic masses after treatment in order to determine whether further courses of chemotherapy should be continued because of residual disease.

Question What complications are associated with this procedure.

Answer This procedure is potentially dangerous because it involves a dissection around the great vessels of the abdomen. In addition to the dangers of haemorrhage due to damage to these vessels, renal vein thrombosis, division of the ureter and chylous ascites have all been described. Large series report complication rates as high as 10 per cent.

Comment Relapse in this patient was followed by chemotherapy and some seven months later by abdominal lymphadenectomy. Seen at intervals one year later his tumour markers have remained so far within normal limits.

26

An Asian female 33 years of age was admitted under the care of a consultant obstetrician in the 25th week of pregnancy having been found on routine examination to be hypertensive.

Previous obstetrical history At the age of 21 she had become pregnant and miscarried. One year later she was again pregnant but in the 37th week she had developed severe pre-eclampsia and labour was induced resulting in a live birth. One year later she spontaneously delivered at full term a baby weighing 3.14 kg but during labour it was noted she was hypertensive, her blood pressure being 140/110 mmHg. Two years later she was again pregnant and was again noted to be hypertensive. Intrauterine death occurred at 32 weeks resulting in a stillbirth. Six months later she miscarried early in pregnancy. Three years later during her sixth pregnancy it was noted that her blood pressure was extremely unstable so that at term she was delivered by Caesarean section. Immediately following delivery her blood pressure was noted to be 165/130 mmHg. Two years later although mildly hypertensive during the later part of her pregnancy she delivered spontaneously at the 39th week. Shortly after this birth she had been referred to a physician, numerous measurements of her blood pressure were taken but all had proved to be normal and no further action had been taken.

In the first trimester of her eighth pregnancy she was again found to be hypertensive and despite the absence of physical signs it was decided that she must be investigated.

Social history The lady was a Muslim, married to a Muslim. She spoke no English and her husband's knowledge was such that communication required the presence of an interpreter.

Question What would you consider to be the probable organic cause of the intermittent hypertension.

Answer This history is suggestive of a phaeochromocytoma particularly in view of the finding that on at least one occasion when the patient was not pregnant she had been found to be hypertensive.

Question In what percentage of hypertensive patients is a phaeochromocytoma the underlying cause.

Answer It has been estimated that a phaeochromocytoma is present in 0.5 per cent of all hypertensives but the majority remain undiagnosed.

Question Is phaeochromocytoma associated with a high fetal and maternal mortality.

Answer Yes. In some recorded series a maternal mortality as high as 50 per cent has been reported, the major causes of death being pulmonary oedema, cerebral haemorrhage and cardiovascular collapse.

Question What are the other causes of hormonal hypertension.

Answer

1 Cushing's disease or syndrome.

2 Primary aldosteronism, first described by Conn in 1954.

3 The excessive production of angiotensin caused either by renal artery stenosis from whatever cause or localized intrinsic renal disease.

Question What is the cause of hypertension in Cushing's disease.

Answer The excessive production of ACTH by the basophil tumour of the pituitary stimulates the excessive production of cortisol and other hormones by the adrenal cortex. It seems probable that together these hormones act through mineralocorticoid receptors to provoke a membrane response in the cation pump which is sodium-dependent. The increased intracellular cationic content of the arterioles potentiates the pressor activity of catecholamines causing an exaggerated contraction of actinomycin and hence hypertension.

Question What is the chief difference between Cushing's disease and Cushing's syndrome.

Answer In Cushing's disease the excessive output of cortisol can be controlled by the administration of dexamethasone which suppresses ACTH secretion.

Question What is the cause of hypertension in Conn's syndrome.

Answer The excessive production of aldosterone by adrenal cortical hyperplasia or tumour causes sodium retention.

Question When was the association between paroxysmal hypertension and phaeochromocytoma first described.

Answer By Frankel in 1886.

Question What does the term phaeochromocytoma mean.

Answer Characteristically these tumours when fixed in bichromate solution become brown due to the stain being taken up by granules in the tumour cells. This reaction is supposed to confirm that the granules contain or consist of catecholamines.

Question To what system of cells do those of the adrenal medulla belong.

Answer The neuroendocrine ADUP system (see Viva 8).

Question Do extra adrenal sites of chromaffin tumours exist.

Answer Yes. Most frequently in childhood hence the greater frequency of both synchronous and metachronous chromaffin tumours before puberty.

Question What extra adrenal sites of adrenal medullary tissue persist beyond childhood.

Answer The carotid body, the glomus jugulare and the aortic body.

Question What tumours other than phaeochromocytoma can occur in the adrenal medulla.

Answer Neuroblastoma and sympathicoblastoma composed of embryonic nerve cells or neuroblasts and ganglioneuroma which are simple tumours containing ganglionic nerve cells and nerve fibres.

Question What are the chief catecholamines produced by the adrenal medulla.

Answer

1 Dopamine. This compound was, until recently, thought to be important only as a precursor of noradrenaline and adrenaline. It has, however, been recently recognized that it plays an important role in the regulation of the splanchnic and renal blood flow.

2 Noradrenaline. This is the chief neurohumoral transmitter agent of the adrenergic fibres of the autonomic nervous system. Both α and β-adrenoreceptors are responsive to its presence.

3 Adrenaline. The chief role of the hormone in the intact animal is on the intermediary metabolism, the stimulation of cAMP by the hormone increasing glycogenolysis and lipolysis. It also acts on the receptors of the heart, mediating an increase in cardiac rate and output with dilatation of the coronary arteries, on the β-receptors of the bronchial muscle causing relaxation and in addition it causes a redistribution of blood from the skin and intestinal vessels to the brain, heart and skeletal muscles.

Normally, phaeochromocytoma secrete much greater quantities of noradrenaline than adrenaline.

Question What other hormone may be elaborated in the adrenal medulla.

Answer Vasoactive intestinal polypeptide (VIP) giving rise to the diarrhoeogenic syndrome.

Question Where, other than in the adrenal medulla, may phaeochromocytomata be found.

Answer Elsewhere in the retroperitoneal area, in the mediastinum, the neck and very rarely in the bladder, the wall of the heart or within the skull.

Question What is the commonest site in which phaeochromocytomata develop.

Answer Ninety-nine per cent of all phaeochromocytomata develop in the abdomen, of which 80 per cent are in the adrenals. In approximately one-fifth of all patients two or more tumours are present, either in the adrenals or elsewhere.

Question Are phaeochromocytoma sporadic or familial tumours.

Answer Ninety-five per cent are sporadic. When a familial genetic component is present approximately 70 per cent are bilateral and the tumours present in the second and third decades. In the majority of familial tumours the presence of phaeochromocytoma is merely one facet of the multiple endocrine adenopathy syndrome, type II A and B. Type IIA, first described by Sippel in 1961, affects the two sexes equally and consists of bilateral medullary carcinoma of the thyroid with a phaeochromocytoma involving one or both adrenal glands. In addition, hyperplasia of the parathyroid glands may be present. This may be due to the same genetic defect or it may be caused by the secretion of thyrocalcitonin from the medullary carcinoma. The much rarer type IIB syndrome is associated with bilateral medullary carcinomata in the thyroid, phaeochromocytoma and multiple true neuromata. These must be distinguished from the neurofibromata found in von Recklinghausen's disease or Schwann cell tumours that may also be associated with phaeochromocytoma. The neuromata are multiple, small subcutaneous or submucosal, lying in the eyelids, tongue and buccal mucosa.

Phaeochromocytomata also occur in association with neuroecto-dermal dysplasias which include von Recklinghausen's disease, tuberous sclerosis, Sturge-Webber's syndrome and Lindau-von Heppel disease.

Question What is the Sturge-Webber syndrome.

Answer A syndrome characteristically associated with fits, mental defect and a facial naevus. The condition is due to a capillary venous mal-formation which usually affects the parieto-occipital region of the brain. Frequently the condition presents in the first decade of life and the diagnosis is suggested by the presence of the facial naevus.

Question What is Lindau-von Heppel disease.

Answer An association of haemoglioblastoma in one cerebellar hemi-sphere associated with cysts in the liver and pancreas, renal tumours and angioma of the retina.

Question What is von Recklinghausen's syndrome.

Answer This is a familial disease inherited as an autosomal dominant although occasional sporadic cases occur. The small nerves of the skin, large peripheral nerves, major nerve trunks and plexuses, spinal nerve roots and ganglia, cranial nerves and autonomic nerves may be affected. The neurofibromata which develop at these sites differ from Schwannomata in that they are less well defined, not encapsu-lated and are an integral part of the nerve. The tumours are pale and may be soft and gelatinous. Histologically the tumour is composed of a proliferation of nerve sheath cells, mainly of Schwann cell origin though often resembling fibroblasts.

In von Recklinghausen's disease irregular, often large, brown pig-mental spots or patches, the café au lait spots, are present on the skin of the trunk or limbs, some of dermatomal distribution. The involvement of the nerves to the skin results in dermal nodules of varying size. In some patients the central nervous system is involved and meningiomata, gliomata of the optic nerve or brain may be present. Phaeochromocytomata are commoner in this disease than in the general population.

Question What are the common symptoms associated with phaeochromocytoma.

Answer The following symptoms in order of frequency are most commonly found in the adult:

1 Persistent hypertension, 65 per cent.
2 Paroxysmal hypertension, 30 per cent.
3 Headache, 80 per cent.
4 Sweating, 70 per cent.
5 Palpitations, 60 per cent.
6 Nervousness, 60 per cent.
7 Tremor, 40 per cent.
8 Nausea, weakness and fatigue, 30 per cent.
9 Weight loss, 15 per cent.

Whilst some of these symptoms obviously suggest the presence of a phaeochromocytoma others suggest the presence of hyperthyroidism or a functional disorder.

Comment In this patient the hypertensive element of her disease had remained transient for many years and its association with pregnancy appears to have led her medical advisers to believe that she was suffering from toxaemia of pregnancy especially as following the birth of her fourth live full term baby she was found to have a normal blood pressure on several occasions.

Question What physical signs, other than hypertension, may be present.

Answer No physical signs are usually present. However, palpitation over the tumour may elicit a rise in blood pressure.

Question What is the underlying cause of the symptoms associated with a phaeochromocytoma.

Answer Few symptoms are ever directly related to the tumour itself although occasionally haemorrhage into the tumour may provoke a complaint of sudden unilateral or bilateral loin pain depending upon whether unilateral or bilateral tumours are present. The major cause, therefore, of the symptoms found in patients suffering from a phaeochromocytoma is the increased production of catecholamines. These hormones and their metabolic products may be detected in the tumour itself, the plasma or the urine.

Normally the episodic release of massive amounts of catecholamines produces severe hypertension, headaches, sweating, tachycardia, pallor and anxiety. Such episodes may terminate in sweating and extreme weakness and indeed in this patient such a transient episode did occur in her eighth pregnancy even though the diagnosis had been made and her blood pressure had apparently been adequately controlled by phenoxybenzamine and propanolol.

Question What tests are required to confirm the clinical diagnosis.

Answer The chief diagnostic test is the estimation of the catecholamines and their metabolites in the blood and urine.

In addition a glucose tolerance test is normally performed to exclude diabetes mellitus since hyperglycaemia is commonly found in this conditions and the thyroid hormone levels are estimated to exclude thyrotoxicosis because many of the symptoms described, excluding hypertension, may occur in severely thyrotoxic patients.

Question What are the normal values for the urinary excretion of catecholamines per day.

Answer

Noradrenaline 0.12–0.7 mmols.

Adrenaline 0.04–0.25 mmols.

Dopamine 0.8–3.0 mmols.

Question What is the normal value for the urinary excretion of hydroxymethyl mandelic acid (HMMA).

Answer 2.0–7.0 mg/day.

Comment In this patient the excretion free catecholamines were increased by a factor of 4, noradrenaline by a factor of 6–7, the adrenaline levels were normal, the dopamine levels were slightly increased and the HMMA was grossly increased.

Question What is HMMA.

Answer Hydroxymethyl mandelic acid, the chief breakdown products of the catecholamines normally found in the urine.

Question How would you localize the position of a phaeochromocytoma.

Answer A variety of investigations are available but if CAT is available this is superior to any other method. Ultrasonography which is also a noninvasive technique is of limited value since tumours less than 3 cm in diameter cannot be identified by this means. Some tumours are hypervascular and can be identified by arteriography but this method is now seldom used.

Some indication of the site may be gained from the hormonal levels, e.g. the ratio of noradrenaline to adrenaline. The N-methylating enzyme for the conversion of noradrenaline to adrenaline is predominantly found in the adrenal medulla and organ of Zuckerkandl.

Therefore, when adrenaline constitutes more than 20 per cent of the total catecholamines in the urine the tumour is almost invariably present in one of these two sites. When noradrenaline alone is increased, as in this patient, the tumour will probably be present in the adrenal or possibly some other intra-abdominal site.

A further screening test is the use of an MIGT scan, this compound being taken up by active chromaffin tissue. Labelled with ^{131}I it can be used to scan the abdomen and thorax for extramedullary sites of actively secreting chromaffin tissue.

Comment This patient was admitted to an obstetrical unit at the 25th week of pregnancy. She was clinically well except that she was grossly obese. Her blood pressure was 150/106 mmHg.

Question How should such a patient be treated.

Answer The blood pressure should be controlled by the administration of an α-adrenergic blocking agent. Two are commonly used, phentolamine mesylate BP (Rogitine, Ciba) and phenoxybenzamine hydrochloride BP (Dibenyline, Smith, Kline and French). Both these drugs have a direct vasodilator effect on all muscular-walled vessels as well as producing α-adrenergic blocking. Both, therefore, abolish vasoconstriction and reduce the blood pressure. However, phentolamine is short acting, the blood pressure returning to normal within 3–4 hours whereas phenoxybenzamine has a much longer action. As the blood pressure falls, however, due to the α-blockage the unopposed β-receptors cause tachycardia and possibly cardiac arrhythmia and the α-blocking agent propranolol BP (Inderal, ICI) is required.

Comment This patient required phenoxybenzamine 30 mg bd and propranolol 20 mg qds to control her blood pressure. However, at the 35th week of pregnancy her diastolic blood pressure began to rise and she became apathetic and listless. In addition two further significant factors developed.

1 The serial 24 hour urinary oestriols level began to fall.
2 Cardiotochographs showed a suspiciously flat pattern.

Question What is the significance of the fall in oestriol levels.

Answer The fall indicates placento-fetal distress.

Question What is cardiotochography.

Answer Cardiotochography is a simultaneous measurement of the fetal ECG and uterine contractions. Normally the fetal heart rate rises during a uterine contraction and falls on relaxation. Any alteration in this pattern suggests the onset of fetal distress.

Comment As a result of these findings an immediate Caesarean section was performed, the baby, weighing 2.5 kg, was delivered through a uterine incision with forceps rather than by fundal pressure. During induction the blood pressure rose to 200/100 mmHg despite the administration of phenotalamine and glyceryltrinitrate. However, within 6 hours the blood pressure had fallen to between 160/100 and 140/80 mmHg and the patient made an uninterrupted immediate recovery being maintained on phenoxybenzamine 20 mg orally bd and propranolol 20 mg qds.

Immediately following recovery attention was turned to the treatment of the phaeochromocytoma.

Question What is the definitive treatment of phaeochromocytoma.

Answer Following diagnosis, localization and pretreatment with α- and β-blocking agents the correct treatment is excision if this is possible. Normally only the relatively rare malignant tumour will not be amenable to surgical excision.

Question Why is medical pretreatment necessary.

Answer Because surgical interference normally provokes the release of large amounts of catecholamines which may precipitate a fatal cardiac arrythmia.

Question What drugs cause the release of catecholamines.

Answer Several drugs and several anaesthetic agents. Indeed in the past histamine or tyramine were used to provoke hypertension in an attempt to establish the diagnosis. Tyramine unlike histamine has a direct action on sympathetic tissue and its intravenous administration causes a steep rise in blood pressure which once attained lasts for 2–3 minutes. These tests are now obsolete.

Question Can circulatory collapse complicate the treatment of a phaeochromocytoma.

Answer Yes. Circulatory collapse may be introgenically induced by the overadministration of drugs such as phentolamine or it may be due to a sudden expansion of the vascular bed following removal of the tumour.

Comment Three weeks post-partum. This patient was admitted for the removal of a right sided phaeochromocytoma which had been identified by four methods:

1 Raised urinary catecholamine levels.

2 Ultrasonography which had identified a suprarenal tumour approximately 9 cm in diameter during pregnancy.
3 CAT which demonstrated no further tumour sites.
4 An MIGT radio-isotope study.

Question What is regarded as an important step in the operation.
Answer Early control of the blood supply to reduce the escape of catecholamines into the peripheral circulation.

Comment Prior to induction of anaesthesia the blood pressure was 130/90 mmHg. A left radial arterial line was inserted, a central venous line and ECG contacts were applied. Immediately following induction the systolic blood pressure rose from 130 mmHg to 200 mmHg and was almost immediately brought under control by the injection of 5 mg of phentolamine, a further rise occurring as the incision was made. Thereafter manipulation of the tumour was followed by further episodes of hypertension with an abrupt fall in both the systolic and diastolic to 80/60 mmHg as the tumour was removed.

At the time of skin closure and extubation the patient's blood presure was recorded as 140/100 mmHg. The patient was transferred to the intensive care ward with orders to receive 1 litre of Hartmann's solution eight hourly and 2 units of whole blood. Seven hours after operation a precipitous fall in blood pressure occurred, the blood pressure falling to 80/60 mmHg. Measurement of the P_{O_2} and P_{CO_2} at this time showed the former to be 4.4 and the latter 6.4, this on an O_2 flow delivered by a Hudson mask of 15 litres with the pH of 7.3. The patient was immediately intubated and ventilation begun. A rapid infusion of plasma protein fraction commenced, 1.2 litres being given over the following seven hours during which time the blood pressure rose to 130/80 mmHg.

Question What is plasma protein fraction.
Answer PPF is composed of 90 per cent albumin. It contains no fibrinogen or antibodies and is used to expand the circulating intravascular space.

Comment As the arterial blood pressure returned to normal the slow infusion of nitroprusside was commenced.

Question What is the action of nitroprusside.
Answer Nitroprusside is an arterial vasodilator somewhat difficult to control and producing severe toxic breakdown products.

Comment Some seven hours later repeated gas studies showed the P_{O_2} to be 4.5 and the pH 7.49. However, seven hours later a further, but less severe, fall in blood pressure occurred, the arterial pressure falling to 100/60 mmHg. The infusion of nitroprusside was, therefore, terminated and a further infusion of 400 ml of PPF given together with dextrose/saline. Six hours later the patient was breathing spontaneously and two hours later still she was extubated. No further problems occurred, her blood gases remained within normal limits breathing 40 per cent oxygen administered by means of a Hudson mask. She made an uninterrupted recovery thereafter.

Pathological examination of the specimen revealed that extensive necrosis, haemorrhage and cystic degeneration had occurred in the tumour which gave a strongly positive chromaffin reaction. There was no evidence of malignancy.

27

A Caucasian female aged 26 was admitted complaining of:
1 Five weeks history of sweating.
2 Anxiety.
3 Palpitation.
4 Tremor.
5 Swelling in the neck.
6 Loss of 7 kilograms in weight.

Previous history Nil of note.

Family history Negative. Her mother and father were alive and well, as were her brother and her two children.

Physical examination

> *Cardiovascular system* P.R. 135. P.B. 160/70. Heart sounds normal.
>
> *Central nervous system* Very anxious woman. Pronounced fine tremor of both hands which were both sweaty and warm. All peripheral reflexes were exaggerated.

Specific examination of the neck revealed a soft symmetrical goitre, a bruit was present over the swelling.

Specific examination of the eyes revealed obvious lid lag, and the suggestion of a left sided proptosis.

Locomotive system No wasting but gross weakness of the proximal muscles of the shoulder girdle. No evidence of arthropathy.

Question What is the presumptive diagnosis.

Answer Primary thyrotoxicosis.

Question In the absence of an enlarged thyroid and the presence of eye signs what other conditions may present with similar symptoms.

Answer
1 An anxiety state.
2 Phaeochromocytoma.

Question What tests are now used to establish the diagnosis of thyrotoxicosis.

Answer Measurement of the T_4 and T_3 values together with the Thyroid Hormone Distribution Index and the Free T_4 index.

Question What are the normal values for these various parameters.

Answer
T_4: 60–140 nmol l^{-1}
T_3: 1.6–3.0 nmol l^{-1}
THDI: 1.2–2.0
Free T_4 index: 1.1–2.7

Comment This patient presented in 1972 at which time these investigations listed were not available to us.

Question What alternative investigations can be used to establish the diagnosis of thyrotoxicosis.

Answer

1 The protein bound iodine. This test was the earliest method routinely used in clinical practice to estimate the concentration of thyroid hormone in the blood. The test measures the total quantity of iodine precipitable with the serum proteins. In the absence of iodine contamination it measures the concentration of T_4 which accounts for approximately 90 per cent of the protein bound iodine. T_3 and other naturally occurring iodine containing compounds precipitable with proteins account for the remaining 10 per cent. The normal range is 4–8 μg I/dl of serum.

Comment In this patient the PBI was 19 μg I/dl.

2 Thyroid uptake of ^{131}I (RAIU). A dose of between 5 and 15 μCi of ^{131}I was given orally and at suitable intervals of time the thyroid content of ^{131}I was determined by a suitable detector. In general the range of normal values is between 5 and 30 per cent.

Comment In this patient ^{131}I uptake was 78 per cent. Both these tests indicated that the patient despite the short history was severely thyrotoxic.

Question What drug will rapidly control the symptoms of thyrotoxicosis without affecting the disease itself.

Answer Propanalol. This drug is a β-adrenoceptor blocking agent. It, together with similar drugs, competitively inhibits the effects of catecholamines at β-adrenergic receptor sites. The principle effect of this drug is to reduce cardiac activity by preventing β-receptor stimulation but the drug also produces symptomatic relief of the catecholamine-provoked tremor in anxiety and hyperthyroidism.

Question What are the contraindications to the use of the drug.

Answer Bronchospasm, sinus bradycardia, heart block and metabolic acidosis.

Comment This patient was discharged home on propranolol 10 mg tds and carbimazole 15 mg qds.

Question What drugs are specifically used to bring the toxic condition itself under control.

Answer Carbimazole and potassium perchlorate.

Question How do these drugs act.

Answer Carbimazole acts by interfering with the incorporation of iodide into thyroglobulin in the thyroid gland and, therefore, reduces the synthesis of tri-iodothyronine and thyroxine. Potassium perchlorate acts by suppressing the uptake of iodine by the thyroid gland.

Normally carbimazole is the drug of choice and perchlorate is only used if this drug proves to be toxic.

Question What is the most serious effect of both drugs.

Answer Agranulocytosis.

Question What is the cause of Graves disease.

Answer The precise cause is unknown. The following factors appear to be of aetiological significance. There is a hereditary background since:

1 (a) The disease may appear in successive generations.

(b) There is a significant increase in incidence among twins.

2 In the white population the inherited predisposition to Graves disease is associated with a HLA-B8 histoincompatibility antigen present in the leucocytes.

Question What features of Graves disease imply that an underlying immune mechanism is present.

Answer

1 There is a general hypertrophy of the lymphoid system.

2 Focal collections of lymphoid tissue occur within the gland itself.

3 Graves disease, thyroiditis and myxoedema often occur in families, patients progressing from one disease to another. Several other autoimmune diseases are associated with these three conditions.

4 Antibodies directed against thyroglobulin and thyroid micro-somal antigen are present in many patients suffering from these conditions and in their relations.

Thus 86 per cent of patients presenting with untreated thyrotoxicosis have circulating antimicrosomal antibodies and 50 per cent anti-thyroglobulin antibodies.

5 In addition to circulating antibodies patients suffering from Graves disease also have gammaglobulin thyroid stimulators in their serum.

Question How can the development of myxoedema in a patient treated with carbimazole be avoided.

Answer By the simultaneous administration of 0.1 mg L-thyroxine tds.

Comment This patient, who was extremely anxious, was kept on the treatment already described together with diazepam 3 mg tds for six months and although at this time she appeared to be euthyroid her goitre had enlarged, the lid lag persisted, some progression of her exophthalmos had occurred and she was complaining of intermittent difficulty in swallowing.

Question What is the cause of lid lag (von Graefe's sign).

Answer Sympathetic overactivity resulting in contraction of the levator palpebrae superiores.

This sign is often associated with infrequent blinking, Stellway's sign.

Question What are the symptoms and signs of exophthalmos.

Answer The common symptoms are: epiphora, eye pain, irritation, grittiness, photophobia and lacrimation. The signs are:

1 Oedema of the lids.

2 Erythema.

3 Chemosis.

4 Protrusion of the globe. Normally the anterior border of the cornea does not protrude more than 18 mm beyond the lateral margin of the orbit.

5 Infiltration of the extra-ocular muscles. The extra-ocular muscles become infiltrated and enlarged. In severe exophthalmos the insertion of the swollen lateral rectus is often visible as a beefy red area at the outer canthus when the eye is turned medially.

6 Paralysis, upward gaze is the first and most severely affected, followed by lack of convergence and oculomotor paralysis.

7 Ultimately fibrosis of the extra-ocular muscles leads to a permanent fixed strabismus.

8 Damage to the optic nerve.

Question What is the pathological cause of endocrine exopthalmos.

Answer A gross increase in bulk of the external ocular muscles together with oedema and lymphoid infiltration of the orbital fat.

Question What changes occur in the extra-ocular muscles.

Answer

1 The muscles lose their striations.

2 Nuclei proliferate.

3 Foci of degeneration appear.

4 The muscles are infiltrated with lymphocytes and plasma cells.

Question What is the cause.

Answer The condition is probably an immune response.

Question What is the temporal relationship between the extraocular and ocular signs of Graves disease.

Answer Extremely variable.

Question How would you differentiate the exophthalmos of Graves disease from other causes of exophthalmos.

Answer The plain X-ray of the orbits is normal and the CT scan shows muscle enlargement.

Question If a CT scan is not available how would you distinguish the exophthalmos of Graves disease from other causes.

Answer If the exophthalmos is unilateral a distinction may be impossible without exploration of the orbit. If the exophthalmos is bilateral orbital ultrasonography may assist. Unfortunately hormonal tests of thyroid function are not always helpful since the levels of circulating T_4 and T_3 may be normal. A positive microsomal antibody test, although not conclusive proof that the exophthalmos is of hormonal origin does prove that autoimmune thyroid disease is present.

Question What simple measures may control the ophthalmopathy of Graves disease.

Answer

1 Control of the thyrotoxic state.
2 0.5% methylcellulose eye drops.
3 Tinted glasses to diminish the photophobia.
4 If there is difficulty in closing the eyes at night taping the eyelids may be useful.
5 When diplopia is present an occluding lens can be helpful.

Question Does control of the thyrotoxicosis necessarily improve the exophthalmos.

Answer It is never wise to give the patient an absolute guarantee that control of the toxic state will necessarily lead to absolute cure. However, in the majority of patients improvement will occur.

Question Are corticosteroids useful in the treatment of this condition.

Answer Yes. Local corticosteroids may combat some of the irritative phenomena but they reduce normal resistance of the cornea to the herpes simplex virus. In severe progressive exophthalmos to prevent optic neuritis developing large doses of prednisone, up to 200 mg a day may be effective. Such high doses should be used only for short periods and when a response has been obtained the dose should be rapidly reduced.

Question What other medical regimes have been described.

Answer The use of immune suppressant drugs such as azathiaprine and cyclophosphamide. These drugs produce variable results.

Question What percentage of patients suffering from 'endocrine' exophthalmos develop malignant exophthalmos.

Answer Very few, 2–3 per cent.

Question If corneal ulceration develops what treatment is required, assuming medical treatment fails.

Answer Orbital decompression. This can be achieved in a variety of ways. The most radical method is the Naffiger operation in which the bony roof of the orbit is excised after access has been gained by means of a frontal bone flap.

Question What is an occasional side effect of Naffziger's operation.

Answer A pulsating eye.

Comment Because the patient continued to feel unwell and complained of difficulty in swallowing she was referred for surgery.

Question In a view of the size of the thyroid gland and the bruit, is Lugol's iodine indicated in the pre-operative preparation of the patient.

Answer No. In the past it was thought that the administration of iodine decreased the vascularity of a toxic gland. Recently reported investigations show that this is not so.

Question What further investigations may provide useful information prior to surgery.

Answer

1 A plain X-ray of the neck and superior mediastinum. This will show the presence or absence of:

(a) tracheal compression.

(b) retrosternal enlargement.

(c) calcification.

2 Antibody levels. The presence of antithyroid and antimicrosomal antibodies indicates the probable development of myxoedema as a long term complication of thyroidectomy.

3 Examination of the cords. Absence of movement of one or both following surgery indicates recurrent laryngeal nerve damage.

Comment In this case microsomal antibodies were present on several examinations.

A subtotal thyroidectomy was performed with difficulty because of the size and extreme vascularity of the gland.

Question Should the recurrent laryngeal nerve be identified.

Answer Yes. It is, however, not sufficient to identify only a small section of the nerve. The whole length of the nerve from its entrance into the neck to its exit into the larynx should be traced.

Question What arteries are divided during the performance of a subtotal thyroidectomy.

Answer The superior thyroid artery, a branch of the external carotid artery. The tracheal vessels which enter the gland from the tracheal area. The inferior thyroid artery, a branch of the thyrocervical trunk. This vessel is not divided but usually ligated in continuity. Some surgeons suggest that the individual branches of this artery should be divided distal to the site of the parathyroid glands in order to preserve their blood supply.

Question What other nerve is endangered when performing a subtotal thyroidectomy.

Answer The external branch of the superior laryngeal nerve which innervates the cricothyroid muscle. These nerves lie close to the vascular pedicles of the superior poles of the gland intimately related in 20 per cent of cases to the superior thyroid vessels.

Question What are the chief immediate complications of thyroidectomy.

Answer

1   Haemorrhage.

2   Thyroid crisis or storm, normally only occurring in patients who have been incompletely controlled prior to surgery.

3   Recurrent laryngeal nerve damage. Damage may be unilateral, bilateral, temporary or permanent. Damage to one recurrent laryngeal nerve results in a cord permanently abducted in a position 3.4 mm from the midline. In addition the cord becomes flaccid. The functional result may be a temporary inability to phonate followed by gradual improvement as the cord tends to become spastic. If injured by excessive traction during the course of surgery function normally returns within six months. When no improvement of phonation has occurred at the end of one year the affected cord should be injected with teflon.

4   Hypoparathyroidism. This may result either from devascularization or excision of the glands. This complication occurs in approximately one per cent of all patients in whom a subtotal thyroidectomy is performed. The clinical manifestions of hypoparathyroidism almost invariably occur within one week of the operation and chiefly consist of circumoral numbness, tingling and anxiety. Tetany affects the peripheral muscles leading to the appearance of carpopedal spasm and the typical appearance of the 'obstetrical hand'. Convulsions and psychoses may develop and long term untreated hypocalcaemia leads to cataract formation.

Comment The histological appearances of the excised gland were typical of primary thyrotoxicosis. The thyroid acini were variable in size and contained scanty colloid. The columnar cells lining the acini showed areas of papillary infolding. There was no evidence of lymphoid infiltration.

The thyroidectomy was extremely difficult due to the great vascularity of the gland. On the fourth post-operative day the patient developed circumoral numbness and examination showed the presence of positive Chvostek and Trousseau's signs.

Question What is Chvostek's sign.

Answer Twitching of the facial muscles on tapping over the facial nerve in front of the ear.

Question What is Trousseau's sign.

Answer Carpal spasm induced by obliterating the radial pulse by inflating a sphygmomanometer cuff applied to the forearm.

Comment The serum calcium was found to be 1.56 mmol/l.

Question What is the normal range.

Answer 2.25–2.60 mmol/l.

Question How would you treat this patient.

Answer By calcium gluconate infusion, giving at the same time oral calcium and vitamin D_3.

Oral calcium gluconate is supplied by Sandoz as an effervescent tablet, each of which contains calcium lactate gluconate 3.08 g, equivalent to 4.5 g of calcium gluconate which provide 10 mmol (400 mg) of calcium.

This patient received 24 g of calcium gluconate intravenously on the day hypocalcaemia developed together with 20000 units of vitamin D_3 and six tablets of calcium (Sandoz). However, on ceasing the intravenous administration of calcium her symptoms rapidly recurred. The intravenous administration of calcium was, therefore, recommenced, 42 g being given on the following day, in addition to three tablets of calcium (Sandoz) qds and 80000 units of vitamin D_3. After three days the intravenous calcium was stopped and she was discharged home six days later on a regime of vitamin D_3 80000 units daily and calcium (Sandoz) three tablets qds.

Question What is the action of vitamin D_3.

Answer

1   It increases the retention of calcium and phosphate.
2   It controls the mineralization of bone.
3   It allows parathyroid hormone to exert its normal effect on bone.

Comment Within seven months of operation the patient was maintained on 100 000 units of vitamin D_3 and was no longer taking calcium. She was seen at intervals over the following five years.

Twelve years after her initial surgery she returned to out-patients complaining of:

1 Loss of 7 kilograms in weight in two months.
2 Tremor.
3 Anxiety.
4 Palpitations.
5 Swelling in the midline of the neck.

In addition in the 10 days prior to her return to outpatients she had noted:

(a) Nausea.
(b) Anorexia.
(c) Thirst, polyuria and polydyspsia.

Question What do these symptoms suggest.

Answer The first group of symptoms suggest recurrent thyrotoxicosis, the second group the development of hypercalcaemia. The latter being confirmed.

Question What is the accepted recurrence rate of toxicity following sub-total thyroidectomy.

Answer Approximately 5 per cent.

Question Is recurrence of hyperthyroidism 12 years after the initial operation common.

Answer Rare.

Question Explain the development of hypercalcaemia in this patient.

Answer Two factors may be responsible:

1 Patients receiving large doses of vitamin D_3, usually, 50 000 units or more daily may develop hypercalcaemia and hyperphosphataemia.

2 Patients suffering from hyperthyroidism develop hypercalciuria and hyperphosphaturia, often associated with normocalcaemia. However, hypercalcaemia may also occur in severe cases.

The sequence of events is:

1 Increased resorption of bone from the action of the excessive amounts of thyroid hormone.
2 Hypercalcaemia from accelerated bone resorption.
3 Decreased secretion of PTH due to the hypercalcaemia.
4 Compensatory decrease in bone resorption.
5 Compensatory decrease in tubular reabsorption of calcium.
6 Hypercalciuria from decreased tubular reabsorption of calcium.

Comment Figures 27.1 and 27.2 shows the physical appearance of the neck in this patient.

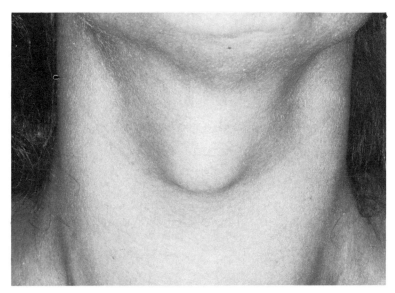

27.1

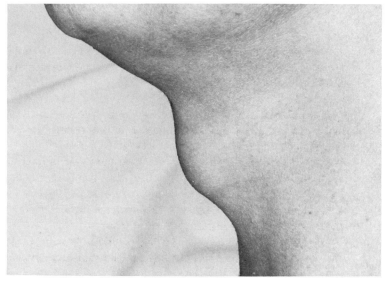

27.2

Question What do these figures show.

Answer A midline swelling.

Question What could this represent.

Answer Hypertrophy and hyperplasia of the pyramidal lobe, possibly causing the recurrence of symptoms.

Question How could this be established.

Answer By performing a thyroid scan. This is shown in Fig. 27.3.

Question What does Fig. 27.3 show.

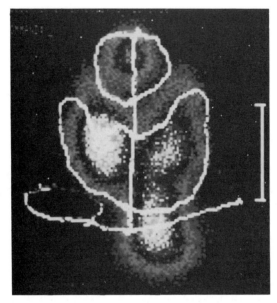

27.3

Answer A central nodule together with almost complete regeneration of both lateral thyroid lobes and a retrosternal extension of the left lobe.

Question Do the appearances indicate the development of a 'hot' nodule.

Answer No. The development of a 'hot' nodule leads to suppression of all remaining thyroid tissue.

Question What, if any, are the contraindications to further surgical treatment.

Answer Caution should be exercised in a patient suffering from recurrent thyrotoxicosis in whom a recurrent laryngeal nerve palsy is already present.

Comment A second thyroidectomy was performed after controlling the patient with sotalol hydrochloride, a non-cardioselective beta-adrenergic blocker, 80 mg tds and carbimazole 15 mg tds.

With great difficulty both the right and left lobes were mobilized and both recurrent laryngeal nerves were identified throughout their course. The right inferior parathyroid gland was identified and three-quarters of each lobe was removed together with the visible midline swelling.

On the day following surgery the patient's voice was weak and examination of the larynx showed that the left cord was paralysed.

Following operation the administration of calcium (Sandoz) and 40000 units of vitamin D_3 was recommenced.

Four months later her voice had returned to normal and examination of the cords showed that both were moving satisfactorily.

Question What alternative treatment could have been offered to this patient.

Answer Treatment with radioactive iodine. Treatment by radioactive iodine is almost inevitably followed by the development of hypothyroidism. Various dose regimes have been described but many depend upon an estimation of thyroid weight which is notoriously difficult to assess. One way of overcoming the danger of myxoedema is to give a relatively large dose of ^{131}I and at the same time administer replacement thyroxine therapy.

Question Other than primary thyrotoxicosis what other causes of hyperthyroidism occur.

Answer

1   Secondary thyrotoxicosis, toxicity in a nodular goitre.

2   A toxic nodule, very rare. This condition results in suppression of the remaining normal thyroid tissue.

3   Thyrotoxicosis factitia, from taking excessive doses of thyroid.

4   Thyrotoxicosis may temporarily occur in thyroiditis.

Comment This patient was last seen nine months following her second operation with no complaints.

Question What are the symptoms of thyroid hormone deficiency.

Answer A large number of symptoms are associated with myxoedema since every system in the body can be affected by lack of circulating thyroid hormone. However, the commonest symptoms include weakness, increasing coarseness and dryness of the skin, lethargy, a sensation of coldness, coarsening of the hair and impairment of memory. There is frequently a gain in weight, loss of hair, hoarseness and anorexia.

Question What are the chief effects of myxoedema in the cardiovascular system.

Answer

1   The cardiac output at rest is decreased because of a reduction in both stroke volume and heart rate reflecting the loss of the inotropic and chronotropic effects of thyroid hormones.

2   The peripheral resistance at rest is increased and the blood volume reduced.

These haemodynamic alterations result in a narrowing of the pulse pressure, a prolongation of the circulation time, and a decrease in blood flow to the tissues. Despite the haemodynamic alterations at rest which resemble those of congestive heart failure, the cardiac output increases and the peripheral resistance decreases normally in response to exercise. Pericardial effusions are common but seldom are of sufficient magnitude as to cause tamponade.

28

A Caucasian male aged 58 years of age was admitted complaining of left-sided renal colic. Seventeen years prior to this admission a right ureterolithotomy had been performed following a similar attack. Analysis of the stone removed at that time had revealed a higher concentration of calcium phosphate than calcium oxalate.

Question What investigations would you perform on this patient.
Answer
1 A plain X-ray of the abdomen followed by an intravenous pyelogram.
2 A biochemical profile.

Question What percentage of renal calculi are radio-opaque.
Answer Over 90 per cent.

Question Which type of stone is radiolucent.
Answer Pure uric acid stone.

Question What other calcific masses may be seen on a plain X-ray of the abdomen.
Answer Calcified costal cartilages, gall stones, phleboliths, fragmentary calcification of the arterial system, uterine fibroids and rarely in the older population of the 'developed' countries lymph nodes affected by *Mycobacterium tuberculosis.*

Question Why must a plain film be taken prior to performing intravenous pyelography.
Answer Because in the presence of reasonable renal function the density of the medium may be sufficient to obscure an opacity.

Question What radiological appearances may be present when the calculus is producing acute obstruction.
Answer A nephrogram due to retention of the medium within the tubular cells and the renal tubules. Follow up films at six hourly intervals will demonstrate the passage of dye into the pelvis and ureter and finally the point of obstruction.

Question How do these radiological findings differ from those of partial obstruction.
Answer In partial obstruction the calyces, pelvis and ureter are dilated down to the site of the obstruction.

Question What are the indications for surgical intervention in a patient proved to have a ureteric calculus causing obstruction of the urinary tract.
Answer
1 A stone greater than 0.5 cm in diameter.

2 Failure of the stone to migrate downwards in the presence of severe symptoms or radiological indications of persistent obstruction.

3 The onset of infection, as judged by a rise in temperature and the presence of an infected urine.

Question How can a ureteric calculus be removed.

Answer

1 If the calculus is in the lower third of the ureter endoscopic methods can be attempted.

2 Proximal to the lower third an open operation should be performed or alternatively, if the technique is available the use of a ureteroscope followed by ultrasonic fragmentation

In this patient the stone was passed spontaneously, the renal colic subsided and interest, therefore, focused on the biochemical profile.

Comment The following are a series of serum calcium levels at different times 2.68, 2.71, 2.65 and 2.74 mmol/l.

Question What is the normal range of serum calcium.

Answer 2.25–2.60 mmol/l.

Question What are the other causes of hypercalcaemia.

Answer Vitamin D intoxication, acute adrenal insufficiency, hyperthyroidism, sarcoidosis, milk-alkali syndrome, neoplasia associated with osseous metastases, multiple myeloma, the acute osteoporosis of disuse. In all these disorders the hypercalcaemia may be associated with hypophosphataemia. The following urinalysis results were obtained from a random 24 hour specimen of urine (volume = 1800 ml).

20.9 mmol Ca in 24 hours. Normal range; 1.25–10 mmol/24 hours.

51.2 mmol PO_4. Normal range; 16–22 mmol/24 hours.

2.4 mmol uric acid. Normal range; 1.2–3.9 mmol/24 hours.

6.2 mmol oxalate. Normal range; 0.2–0.5 mmol/24 hours.

Question What does this biochemical study suggest.

Answer The possibility, in the absence of any underlying cause, of a parathyroid adenoma.

Question Could the excessive urinary calcium excretion be explained in any other way apart from the presence of an underlying cause.

Answer Yes. Idiopathic hypercalciuria is the commonest cause of excessive calcium excretion. However, idiopathic hypercalciuria is not associated with a raised serum calcium. Therefore, either some cause other than primary hyperparathyroidism is present or the patient is suffering from primary hyperparathyroidism.

Question In hyperparathyroidism would you expect the serum PO_4 to be lower than normal.

Answer Yes. In this case, however, the phosphate level was only at the lower end of the normal range measuring 0.82 mmol/l.

Question What study accurately reflects parathyroid activity.

Answer Measurement of the circulating level of PTH. In this patient two assays of the PTH were performed, the first 210 pg/ml was disappointingly low, the second, however, was 500 pg/ml as compared to the normal range of between 125–375 pg/ml.

Question The raised level of PTH now suggests the presence of a parathyroid adenoma. What confirmatory biochemical test can be performed.

Answer Estimate the cAMP (cyclic adenosine 3′,5′-monophosphate).

Question What is the action of cAMP.

Answer cAMP is the primary mediator of the action of PTH. The hormone in this case parathyroid hormone (PTH) is known as the first messenger. This is released from the endocrine gland, the parathyroids, and interacts with receptors on the plasma membrane of the target cell. The interaction between hormone and receptor causes an increase in the activity of the enzyme adenylate cyclase which leads to an increase in the rate of formation of cAMP. This alters certain enzyme activities or other cell processes eliciting a response from the cell characteristic of the action of the particular hormone.

cAMP in cell free and intact cell preparations produces bone resorption stimulating adenylate cyclase activity in both the kidney and bone.

Question What is the unit of measurement of cAMP.

Answer nmol/litre of glomerular filtrate.

Question Why in the urine.

Answer Because cAMP produced by the tubular cells of the kidney appears largely in the urine and only minimally in the plasma. In this case the value obtained was 48.3 nmol/l (normal value 15–40 nmol/l).

Question The diagnosis of a parathyroid adenoma having been established what is the correct treatment.

Answer Exploration of the neck and removal of the tumour.

Question In approximately what percentage of patients is more than one adenoma present.

Answer 20 per cent.

Question What are the effects of parathyroid hormone on bone.

Answer The response of bone to PTH is biphasic. The first or immediate phase beginning within minutes or hours of a rise in the circulating level of PTH depends upon the effect of PTH on bone cell activity, the second depends upon the effect of PTH on the size of active bone cell pools.

Question What is the immediate effect of administering PTH to a parathyroidectomized animal.

Answer Osteocytic and osteoclastic osteolysis are increased due to an increase in the activity of both types of cells and by decreasing bone matrix synthesis through decreasing the activity of osteoblasts.

Question What biochemical changes follow these effects.

Answer The plasma calcium concentration rises together with the urinary excretion of calcium and hydroxyproline. There is also an increase in the rate of conversion of 25 (OH) D_3 to 1,25 (OH)$_2$ D_3 in renal tissue.

Question What later cellular effect follows these effects.

Answer An increasing number of new osteoclasts are formed but if the administration of PTH is continued the enlarged osteoclast pool leads to a secondary increase in the flow of cells into the oestoblast pool, with a resultant increase in bone formation as well as bone resorption. However, resorption is normally greater than formation resulting in the net negative skeletal balance observed in hyperparathyroidism.

Question What is the result of the increased conversion of 25 (OH) D_3 to 1,25 (OH)$_2$ D_3 in the renal tissue.

Answer An increase in calcium absorption from the intestine.

Question In what percentage of patients suffering from hyperparathyroidism is osseous involvement present.

Answer Bone involvement detectable by radiological or bone biopsy studies is only present in about 30 per cent of cases but more sophisticated tests, e.g. using microradiographic techniques and isotope studies show the presence of bone disorder in 60–65 per cent.

Question How does this compare with renal involvement.

Answer Recognizable renal signs or symptoms are present in about 80 per cent of affected individuals. The two occurring together in about 50 per cent of cases.

Question What symptoms does bone involvement cause.

Answer The commonest symptom is vague bone pain regarded by the patient as 'rheumatism'. Progression of the disease may lead to fragility associated with an increased incidence of fractures and the development of bone cysts and so-called 'brown tumours'.

Question What is the fate of bone tumours and bone cysts following parathyroidectomy.

Answer The bone tumours disappear to be replaced by bone but the cysts remain as radiolucent areas.

Question What are the classic radiological signs of hyperparathyroidism.

Answer Resorption of the subperiosteal bone in the metacarpals and phalanges of the fingers, the 'rotten gate post' sign (Fig. 28.1), the ground glass appearance of the skull (Fig. 28.2) and if the teeth are still present the absence of the lamina dura surrounding them.

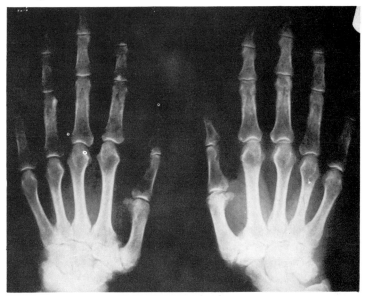

28.1

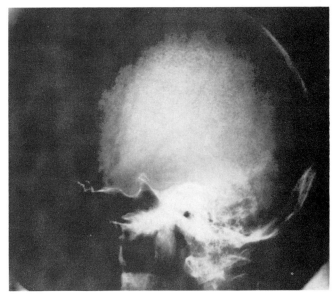

28.2

Question What are the characteristic histological signs of hyperparathyroidism.

Answer There is increased formation and increased resorption of bone and many osteoclasts. There is an increase in the amount of osteoid and an increase in the number of osteoblasts which appear less active than normal. In addition there is a loss of normal trabecular architecture with replacement of lamellar bone by woven bone, this change producing the ground glass appearance of the bone.

Question What is osteoid.

Answer Decreased mineralization of bone, the matrix of the bone being uncalcified. Such bone is weaker than normal hence the production of deformity or fracture under stress.

Question What is osteoid.

Answer Decreased mineralization of bone, the matrix of the bone being uncalcified. Such bone is weaker than normal hence the production of deformity or fracture under stress.

Question What is woven bone and how does it differ from lamellar bone.

Answer The former consists of coarse fibre bundles running in an irregular interlacing pattern through a matrix rich in ground substance. Woven bone is the type of bone laid down in the embryonic skeleton or found in the pathological conditions of Paget's disease, hyperparathyroidism and fibrous dysplasia.

In the course of normal development it is replaced by lamellar bone which is stronger in which the fibre bundles run in parallel sheets, different sheets running in different directions to produce a stratified appearance.

Question Are there any signs specifically associated with hypercalcaemia.

Answer A decrease occurs in the excitability of the neuromuscular apparatus causing muscular weakness of a profound degree in some patients. Calcium phosphate crystals may be deposited in the conjunctiva of the palpebral fissure and band keratitis is common. Metastatic calcification is rare in contrast to the situation in hypervitaminosis D in which it is relatively common.

Question How is a parathyroid adenoma recognized.

Answer In only a very small number of patients is the adenoma within the thyroid itself. Approximately 97 per cent lie outside the thyroid and are almost completely separate from the capsule. They normally contain some fat, have a more uniform appearance than thyroid tissue itself and when not obscured by fat the tumours are dusky red in colour. The trick in identification is to keep the operation field as bloodless as possible. Normal parathyroid glands are approximately $3\times3\times5$ mm. When a parathyroid adenoma is present the remaining glands atrophy making their identification difficult if not impossible. Frozen sections of suspected tissues should be examined before closing the neck.

Question If a parathyroid adenoma has been identified and removed what is the effect.

Answer This depends on the initial presenting symptom. In rare cases the patient suffering from hypercalcaemia may present in coma or with marked aberations of mental function including delusions and hallucinations. In such cases improvement is dramatic. In patients complaining of abdominal pain relief can be expected. In patients suffering from recurrent urinary calculus formation the formation of stones ceases. In patients presenting with bone tumours, resembling osteoclastomata, these disappear to be replaced by normal bone.

29

A male Caucasian age 54 was referred complaining of right calf pain ascending to the thigh after walking approximately 100 yards. The pain was relieved by resting for 2–3 minutes. He had smoked 30 cigarettes a day for some 34 years.

He had never suffered from pain in the chest or spontaneous pain in the legs. Five years previously he had been found to have hypertension on a routine insurance examination and had been treated with mifedipine (Aldalat, Bayer) 10 mg tds.

Examination Inspection revealed a somewhat obese man.

Abdominal examination	Negative.
Cardiovascular system	BP 190/100 mmHg. No other abnormality.
Respiratory system	No abnormality.
Peripheral pulses	Both femoral pulses were palpable and were much weaker than normal. Auscultation revealed a bruit over the right common femoral artery below the inguinal ligament. Both popliteal pulses were present, the right being weaker than the left. Both posterior tibial pulses were present, both very weak. Inspection of the feet revealed that the right foot was slightly bluer than the left. Both feet felt abnormally cold.

Question On what factors does the cutaneous temperature depend.

Answer On the total amount of heat brought to the surface of the body by the blood in the cutaneous vessels and the amount lost through convection, radiation and vaporization.

Question What does the skin colour of the feet reflect.

Answer Skin colour, assuming a normal haemoglobin, reflects the rate of blood flow through the cutaneous vessels. In a normal individual lying in the horizontal position the skin has a slightly pinkish flush. The presence of pallor, cyanosis or rubor indicates some alteration of the local vascular system.

Question What additional simple clinical test will confirm that the circulation has fallen to a critical level in the feet.

Answer Observe the colour changes in the feet on first elevating the lower limbs and then making them dependent.

In a person in whom the peripheral circulation is normal the skin of the feet should continue to remain pink on elevation although perhaps slightly paler. The appearance of pallor indicates a reduced arterial circulation. If the legs are now put into a dependent position the feet should return to their normal pink colour within 10 seconds.

In a patient suffering from arterial insufficiency there is a delay in the reappearance of the normal skin colour for as long as 45 seconds and the change may then be patchy rather than uniform. In addition, in this situation, an intense cyanotic rubor will develop.

Question What is, and how do you perform, the reactive hyperaemia test.

Answer The reactive hyperaemia test measures the response of the peripheral circulation to a period of ischaemia. The limb is drained of blood by elevating it, after which a blood pressure cuff is applied and inflated to a pressure exceeding the systolic blood pressure. Occlusion is maintained for 3 minutes. The cuff is then released. In a normal limb, due to the development of an oxygen debt, reactive hyperaemia spreads from the site of the cuff to the toes in a period of 10–15 seconds, the flush remaining for between 10 and 40 seconds after which it recedes.

When arterial insufficiency is present there is a delay in the appearance of the flush which is also patchy and cyanotic rather than red and the response may take 2–3 minutes to reach the digits and a long delay follows before it completely disappears.

Comment In this patient these simple clinical tests were positive, indicating arterial insufficiency in both limbs.

Previous medical history Six years previously he had complained of bleeding per rectum, together with occasional attacks of intermittent abdominal colic occurring every three months. Investigation revealed third degree haemorrhoids and a Milligan Morgan haemorrhoidectomy was performed.

Four years previously he complained of claudication in the right buttock after walking 300 yards. Examination at that time had revealed a reduced pulse pressure in the right common femoral artery.

A retrograde aortogram was performed via the left common femoral artery. The result is shown in Fig. 29.1.

Question What are the significant findings shown in Fig. 29.1.

Answer

1 A short but severe stenosis of the right common iliac artery just proximal to the origin of the right internal iliac artery.

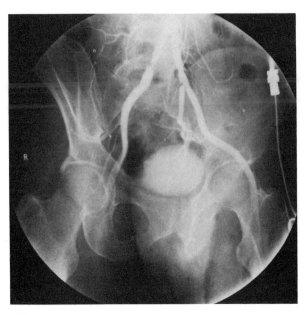

29.1

2 Absence of the right internal iliac artery.

3 A tight stenosis at the origin of the left internal iliac artery.

Question What is the pathological cause of these stenotic lesions.

Answer Atherosclerosis.

Question What are the chief risk factors associated with the development of this condition.

Answer

1 Hypercholesterolaemia.

2 Hypertension.

3 Smoking.

Question What would be the histological appearance of the narrowed segment of the right common iliac artery.

Answer This segment will consist of an atherosclerotic plaque in which extracellular calcium, blood components, cholesterol crystals and glycosaminoglycans are present. This plaque will be exposed to the blood stream because of the loss of the surface endothelium and deep to the deposit the internal elastic lamina and the media will be fragmented. Haemorrhagic areas may also be present deep to the plaque due to rupture of the vasa vasorum.

Comment At this time the patient was offered treatment but in view of the fact that the claudication rarely incapacitated him, he was a clerical worker whose chief hobby was bridge, he declined.

Question Why perform an arteriogram.

Answer To establish the following:

1 The size of the vessel involved.
2 The site of the primary occlusion.
3 The existence of other sites of obstruction in the limb.
4 The condition of the vessel proximal and distal to the main occlusion.
5 The extent of the collateral circulation and the run off vessels.

Question How can the changes in the pulses be calibrated.

Answer By the use of a Doppler probe. A cuff is placed on the limb and inflated, the Doppler probe is then placed over the artery and the cuff slowly deflated. A sound is heard as the low-intensity ultrasonic beam is reflected from the moving column of blood. This is the systolic pressure. It can then be compared with the brachial systolic pressure to produce a pressure index which in a normal person should be unity.

Question What treatment would you have advised in view of the arteriographic findings.

Answer Percutaneous transluminal angioplasty.

Question When was this technique first developed.

Answer PTA was first introduced by Dotter and his colleagues in 1964 who used a coaxial catheter. A further significant development was the introduction by Gruntzig in 1974 of a balloon catheter made of polyvinyl chloride which is given its cylindrical shape during its manufacture. Such a balloon can withstand 3–4 atmospheres and will not take up an hour glass shape when expanding within a stenotic lesion.

Question What is the mechanism by which angioplasty improves flow through a stenotic segment.

Answer The basic mechanism is believed to be stretching of the intima, media and adventitia to such a degree that the intima and media rupture. This results in a permanent widening of the artery which becomes lined by a neointima.

For further information on the use of angioplasty see Viva 30.

Comment In view of the worsening of the patient's condition a further arteriogram was performed using a 5 French Catheter and 37 ml of urografin 370 diluted with normal saline.

Question What does Fig. 29.2 show.

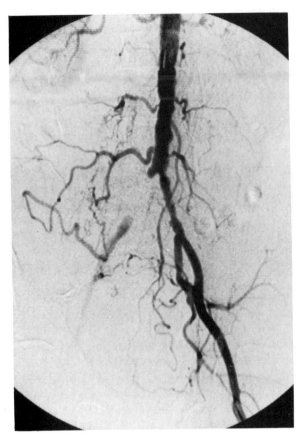

29.2

Answer The chief feature shown is the rapid deterioration in the major
blood vessels. The major findings are:
1   Gross irregularity of the wall of the aorta.
2   Total occlusion of the right common iliac artery from a point just
distal to its origin from the aorta, to a point just proximal to the
origin of the right internal iliac artery.
3   Gross mural irregularity of the left common iliac artery.
4   Stenosis of the origin of the left internal iliac artery.
5   Poor run off down the right external iliac, common and superficial
femoral when compared to the situation in the left leg.
6   The right and left superficial femoral arteries distal to the origin
of both profunda arteries appeared normal.

Question What would you consider are the chief indications for surgical intervention.

Answer

1 Intermittent claudication limiting daily activities.

2 Accelerating intermittent claudication.

3 Ischaemic neuropathy leading to rest pain.

4 Gangrene limited to the toes.

Comment In view of the reduction in the claudication distance and arteriographic evidence of advancing pathology surgical interference was advised.

Question What operation would you consider the most suitable in this patient.

Answer An aorto-femoral Y graft.

Question Assuming that the patient was several years older and quite unfit for an abdominal operation what alternative surgical procedure might be possible.

Answer An axillo-femoral bypass. This can be performed on one side only using a cross over graft from the axillo-femoral graft to the contralateral femoral artery or as a bilateral procedure.

Question In this case what type of anastomoses would you use.

Answer End of graft to side of aorta and ends of the Y graft to the point at which the common femoral divides into the superficial femoral and its profunda branch.

Question What factors adversely affect the outcome of arterial grafts.

Answer

1 Technical operative errors.

2 Inadequate run off.

3 Proximal progression of the disease.

4 When a vein graft is used, stenosis of the graft due to valve cusp stenosis.

5 Infection.

Question What type of graft is suitable for a case such as this.

Answer Knitted Dacron (polyethylene terephthalate). This type of graft must be preclotted before being stitched into position. Newer types of graft have now been manufactured in which this is unnecessary; they are, however, much more expensive (see Viva 30).

Question What vessels must be controlled before clamping the aorta.

Answer The lower end of the aorta and the lumbar arteries, the superficial femoral and the profunda arteries.

Question If possible the common iliac arteries should be left alone. Why.

Answer Because:

    1 They are sometimes bound by periarteritis to the common iliac veins which may cause troublesome bleeding if torn during their dissection.

    2 The hypogastric sympathetic plexus flows across the left iliac artery, division of this plexus causes impotency.

Question How do we expose the common femoral artery.

Answer A vertical incision is made in the line of the mid-inguinal point crossing the groove of the groin and extending for approximately 10 cm below it.

    The incision is deepened until the artery is exposed. The vessel, if not pulsating, is recognized by the small blood vessels in the adventitia. Care should be taken not to damage the long saphenous vein which may be needed at a later date for a bypass graft. Control must be obtained proximally, distally and of the profunda femoris. Smaller unnamed arteries can be temporarily occluded by a double loop of thread.

Question When suturing the graft to the arteries in which direction should the stitch be taken.

Answer From within the artery rather than into the artery. In this way damage to the intima is kept to a minimum.

Question Other than infection what local complication may occur in the groin wounds.

Answer Isolation of the femoral vessels involves division of lymphatic vessels with the result that a collection of lymph may form a pocket in the subcutaneous tissues. This must be aspirated using aseptic precautions in order to prevent sepsis.

Question Assuming that the run off remains satisfactory what is the prognosis of aorto-iliac surgery.

Answer Excellent. Five year patency rates as high as 85 per cent have been reported.

30

A white male, 77 years of age was admitted with the following history. Four days prior to admission whilst trimming his toe nails with scissors the instrument had slipped and cut into the skin of the third right toe. There had been little bleeding and he had, therefore, treated the small penetrating wound with a small gauze dressing. However, four days later he had noted that the skin of the toe pad of the third toe had turned black as also had the skin on the medial aspect of the fourth toe. At that point he had called his own doctor and his acute admission to hospital had been arranged.

Examination on admission revealed the signs already noted above by the patient but in addition the right foot was cold with skin mottling as far proximal as the mid-calf.

Examination of the peripheral pulses; on the right side the common femoral, popliteal and anterior and posterior tibial pulses were absent. On the left side the common femoral was clearly palpable, the popliteal barely so and the anterior and posterior tibial arteries were absent. Other than this his general condition was exceedingly good for a man of such advanced years.

Previous history Ten years prior to admission at 67 years of age he had been referred complaining of intermittent crushing pains in the chest associated with referred pain in the right upper arm. Investigation had revealed a mild degree of hypertension, blood pressure 165/85 and oxyprenalol 40 mg bd, later altered to Atenolol 100 mg daily had been prescribed, together with sublingual glyceryl trinitrate tablets.

Nine years prior to admission he had developed pain in the right buttock and calf, the pain developing after walking some 500 yards relieved by rest.

Six years prior to admission his claudication distance had suddenly fallen to some 200 yards and he was referred to hospital.

Examination at that time had revealed absent pulses in the common femoral artery and beyond but very significantly an iron deficiency anaemia, his haemoglobin on admission being 6.4 g/dl. The serum B_{12} and folate levels were normal. He was investigated, no cause other than severe colonic diverticulosis was found and he was prescribed iron. As the haemoglobin level rose to normal levels his claudication distance increased again to over 500 yards and the frequency of his anginal attacks diminished.

For this reason no further investigation of his vascular system was initiated and he was reviewed at six monthly intervals during which, up to the time of his self-inflicted accidental injury his condition remained stable.

Question At the time of his acute admission what is the clinical diagnosis.

Answer Dry gangrene of the third and fourth toes.

Question What pathological lesion is the underlying cause of this condition.

Answer Obviously from simple clinical examination extensive arterial disease of the right lower extremity is present, extending proximally as far as the aorto-iliac segment, hence the absence of the pulse in the common femoral artery noted some six years prior to admission.

Question Is the cardiac condition related to the condition of the foot.

Answer Not directly but it does indicate that this patient is suffering from generalized atherosclerosis.

Question How does glyceryl trinitrate relieve the pain of angina pectoris.

Answer This drug causes peripheral vasodilatation and hence decreases the venous return to the heart thus reducing the left ventricular volume and the energy expenditure. The degree of relaxation of the coronary arteries is not considered sufficient to appreciably increase the cardiac blood flow directly.

Question In sublingual tablet form how long is it before the drug is effective in relieving cardiac pain.

Answer 2–3 minutes.

Question How long is the effect.

Answer 30–60 minutes.

Question What is the normal dose.

Answer 0.5–1 mg. Sustained action tablets of 2.6, 6.4 and 10 mg are available, to be taken three times a day.

Question What adverse side effects does glyceryl trinitrate cause.

Answer Flushing of the face, dizziness, tachycardia and throbbing headaches.

Question What type of drugs are oxyprenalol and atenolol.

Answer Both are β-blockers but whereas oxyprenalol is classified as non-cardioselective, atenolol is classified as cardioselective.

Question What adverse side effects can be produced by these drugs.

Answer Adverse side effects occur in various systems producing:

1 In the gastrointestinal tract, nausea, vomiting and diarrhoea.

2 In the cardiovascular system, bradycardia, congestive heart failure, heart block and Raynaud's phenomenon.

3 In the central nervous system, fatigue, dizziness, depression, hallucinations, disturbances of sleep and vision.

4 In the respiratory system, bronchospasm.

Question How has the right limb managed to survive for so long.

294

Answer By the development of collateral circulation around the chief areas of disease.

Question Name the chief vessels of the pelvis which serve to provide a collateral circulation across the pelvis from one side to the other.

Answer The lateral sacral, iliolumbar, obturator and internal pudendal arteries are medial branches of the internal iliac artery which serve to connect the two sides of the pelvis.

Question What vessels provide a collateral circulation between the pelvis and the lower extremity.

Answer The lateral branches of the internal iliac artery, i.e. the superior and inferior gluteal arteries which anastomose caudal to the inguinal ligament with the medial and lateral circumflex arteries, branches of the profunda femoris artery.

Question In response to slowly developing arterial obstruction does the collateral circulation tend to be concentrated in few arteries or involve a multiplicity of smaller vessels.

Answer Fewer large, rather than many small in response to the physical laws governing the flow of a liquid through a tube, i.e. Poiseuille's Law.

Question What does the Law of Poiseuille state.

Answer That the velocity of flow of a liquid through a capillary tube varies directly as the pressure and the fourth power of the diameter and inversely as the length of the tube and the coefficient of viscosity. According to this law when the diameter of an artery is doubled, all other factors remaining equal, the flow within it is increased 16 times.

Question What has precipitated the development of gangrene in this patient.

Answer The additional burden placed on the microcirculation by the injury and the associated infection. The repair of the injury requires an increase in the blood supply to the skin which cannot be attained in such an already compromised limb.

Question If no surgical procedure is possible what will be the probable fate of the limb.

Answer Probably slow extension of gangrene followed by the necessity for an above knee amputation. In an individual, 77 years of age, this will probably lead to permanent invalidism.

Question In view of the physical findings what investigation will be of most assistance to the surgeon contemplating direct arterial surgery.

Answer Arteriography using a Seldinger catheter inserted through the left common femoral artery and upwards into the aorta.

Comment In the General Infirmary at Leeds we have a digital vascular imaging (DVI) available.

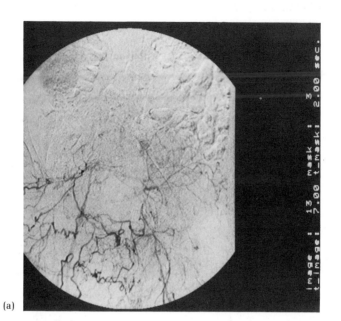

(a)

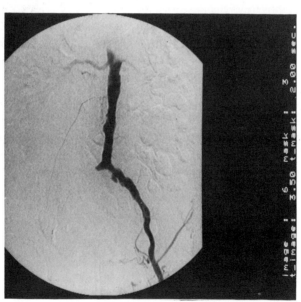

(b)

30.1

Question What, if any, are the advantages of the latter technique over conventional angiographic techniques.

Answer

1　A much smaller cannula can be used thus diminishing the risks associated with direct puncture of a diseased vessel.

2　Much smaller quantities of medium are required to produce adequate imaging, thus reducing the toxic effects associated with iodine. The material used Conray 277 is a non-ionized iodine preparation.

Comment In this case the result of this investigation is shown in Figs 30.1(a), 30.1(b), 30.2, 30.3 and 30.4.

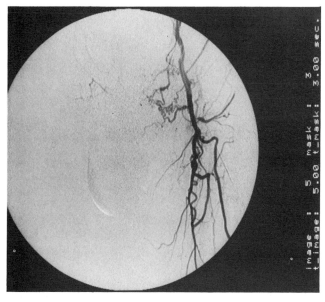

30.2

Question What are the chief findings.

Answer

1　Atheromatous changes in the lower abdominal aorta (Fig. 30.1(a)).

2　Extensive pelvic anastomoses (Fig. 30.1(b)).

On the left side:

   (a) Disease of the common iliac artery (Fig. 30.1(a)).

   (b) Patent external iliac and common femoral arteries (Fig. 30.2).

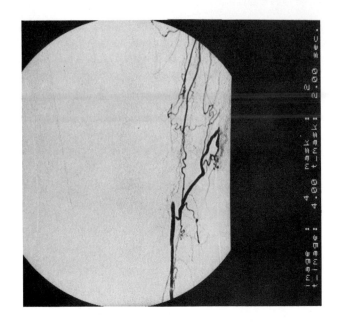

30.3

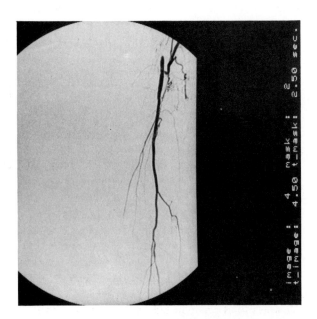

30.4

(c) Occlusion of the upper and middle thirds of the superficial femoral artery. Flow down the thigh being maintained by the profunda femoris, its penetrating branches, and a number of collaterals (Fig. 30.3).

(d) A patent popliteal artery with excellent run off arteries (Fig. 30.4).

3 On the right side, a complete block of the common femoral iliac artery is shown from a point 1 cm distal to the origin of the aorta as also is the blocked external iliac artery. Narrow but patent common femoral and profunda femoris arteries were seen on other films the vessels receiving their supply from the pelvic collaterals. The lower third of the superficial femoral artery was blocked but bridged by collaterals.

Question In view of the above radiological findings is direct intervention indicated.

Answer Yes.

Question What procedure would you consider might be feasible.

Answer Bypass of the blocked area using a Y graft of artificial material.

Question What is the most commonly used material.

Answer Polyethylene terephthalate (Dacron). Dacron grafts are of two types, kitted and woven. The advantage of the woven graft is that the fibres are more tightly packed and, therefore, bleeding through the interstices of the graft is less. All grafts have, however, to be preclotted before stitching *in situ*, except for the Knitted Microvel, Double Velour Graft known as Hemashield which is impregnated with collagen.

Question What is the disadvantage of the last material.

Answer

1 It is expensive.

2 Remaining portions cannot be resterilized for reuse.

Comment In this patient, having obtained control of the aorta and both common femoral arteries a Y graft was inserted, all three anastomoses being end to side, i.e. end of graft to side of blood vessel.

Question Would you give heparin during the course of the operation.

Answer Yes. 5000 units prior to cross clamping the aorta. It is also essential to flush the lower limb vessels with heparin solution before clamping.

Question Would you use anticoagulants following the termination of the operation.

Answer This matter is still debated by vascular surgeons. One recommended regime is the use of subcutaneous heparin 5000 units, three times a day.

Question What material would you use to suture the graft in place.

Answer 7/0 prolene, this material has the advantage of sliding easily through the tissues and is less thrombogenic than multifilamentous materials.

Question What are the major immediate complications of this surgical procedure.

Answer

1   Haemorrhage.

2   Thrombosis.

3   Paralytic ileus.

4   Rarely necrosis of the rectum from division of the inferior mesenteric artery.

In this patient the last complication would certainly not occur since during the initial exploration the inferior mesenteric artery was seen to be occluded.

5   Infection.

Comment Some eight hours after the completion of the operation the left lower limb was showing ischaemic changes from the midthigh distally. One litre of Dextran 70 was given over a period of four hours and some four hours later the mottled changes of pronounced ischaemia had receded to involve only the lower calf and foot. However, after a further period of six hours no obvious improvement had occurred.

Question Why was Dextran 70 administered.

Answer Dextran 70, molecular weight 70000 can be shown *in vitro* to counter the aggregation of red cells and the adhesiveness of platelets. Therefore, on the assumption that thrombus formation or clot had occurred in the left leg the infusion of Dextran could theoretically at least ameliorate the condition.

Question Can any other explanation be advanced to explain the sudden deterioration of the left leg when at the same time the right leg and foot has so obviously improved following operation.

Answer It could be postulated that what we are witnessing is 'steal', the blood finding an easier path down the right side than the left because of the patent common femoral and profunda vessels whereas on the now compromised left side the superficial femoral is blocked in its upper and middle thirds.

Question With established ischaemic changes in the left leg what treatment is now indicated.

Answer Immediate exploration of the lower limb vessels. Reopen the L groin wound. After gaining control of the common femoral, profunda and superficial femoral arteries, perform an arteriotomy below the level of the original end to side Y graft.

Pass a Fogarty catheter down both the common femoral, the superficial femoral and the profunda arteries. Note that since the superficial femoral is blocked in its upper and middle thirds one would not expect the catheter to progress along in this vessel for more than a few centimetres.

Comment From both vessels clot was extruded on withdrawing the catheter. Access to the profunda was gained via a transverse arteriotomy in the Y graft.

Question Is any further surgery necessary.

Answer In this patient it is probably best to circumvent the blocked superficial femoral artery by some form of bypass graft. In this patient a woven Dacron graft was used, performing end to side anastomoses using 5/0 Prolene sutures. The graft was placed within the subsartorial canal and the lower end anastomosed to post-femoral portion of the popliteal artery.

N.B. Other techniques could have been considered. These will be discussed in greater detail in Viva 31. The aim, however, in this patient was to obtain an improved blood flow to the lower limb in the shortest operating time possible, remembering that this patient was 77 years of age and had already had one major operation only 24 hours previously.

Comment The patient did well. The left leg was saved completely; the two gangrenous toes on the right foot were eventually amputated. However, between the first and third post-operative days the patient developed severe oedema of the left leg.

Question Why.

Answer Due to the increased capillary filtration pressure in a limb previously chronically underperfused.

31

A Caucasian male aged 60 was admitted complaining of pain in the right foot together with severe discoloration of the fourth and fifth toes. Apparently he had involuntarily stood on a tube of toothpaste two weeks previously and thereafter felt a dull pain in the foot, which had gradually become worse. The discoloration of the toes had been first noticed four days prior to admission. He admitted to smoking 30 cigarettes a day.

Previous medical history

1   Fifteen years prior to admission he had suffered a mild myocardial infarct.

2   Ten years prior to admission he had been found to suffer from diabetes which had been successfully controlled by diet.

3   Four years prior to admission he had developed intermittent claudication, his walking distance being reduced to between 100–200 yards.

Drug regime His present medication included:

Attenolol 100 mg daily.

Digoxin 250 μg by mouth bd.

Spirolactone 25 mg bd.

Physical examination

Cardiovascular system   BP 210/130 mmHg. Heart rate normal. Rhythm normal.

Peripheral pulses

	Right leg	Left leg
Femoral	−	+
Popliteal	−	−
Anterior tibial	−	−
Posterior tibial	−	−

Inspection of the right foot revealed dry gangrene of the fifth toe extending proximally to the toe cleft together with redness and swelling of the whole of the forefoot.

Respiratory system   No abnormality.

Central nervous system   No abnormality.

Question What is the diagnosis.

Answer Gangrene of the foot associated with gross arteriopathy and diabetes.

Question What are the actions of the various drugs.

Answer

1 Atenolol is a cardioselective β-adrenergic blocking agent with an action similar to propanolol but being cardioselective it is less likely to cause bronchospasm. Its principal effect is to reduce the response of the heart to stress and exercise and to reduce the blood pressure in patients suffering from hypertension. It reduces the incidence of angina pectoris in patients suffering from myocardial ischaemia.

2 Digoxin. This drug is a cardiac glycoside which acts upon the heart by a positive inotropic effect and also by affecting atrioventricular conduction and vagal tone. It is normally used in patients suffering from congestive cardiac failure with the additional administration of a diurectic.

3 Spirolactone is a diuretic whose action is mediated via the inhibition of aldosterone. It acts on the distal portion of the renal tubule increasing sodium and water excretion and reducing potassium excretion. It should not, therefore, be given to patients suffering from hyperkalaemia or renal failure.

Question What urgent investigations are required.

Answer

1 Full blood count.

2 Fasting blood sugar.

3 Bacteriology of the necrotic area.

Comment

1 The full blood count showed the Hb to be 16.5 g/dl and the total nucleated cell to be 12.5×10^9/l, granulocytes 82.3%.

2 Fasting blood sugar 9.070 mmol/l (N value 3.3–5.6 mmol/l).

3 Streptococcus haemolytic grew from a swab taken from toes.

Question What treatment is necessary.

Answer

1 Control the infection. In this case benzylpenicillin sodium BP 600 mg every four hours was given.

2 Control the hyperglycaemia. In this patient the drug glibenclamide 5 mg daily was commenced. This drug is an oral sulphonylurea with similar actions and uses to chlorpropamide.

Question What other biochemical tests might be helpful.

Answer Estimation of the total cholesterol and triglycerides. In this patient the results of both were within normal limits. Total cholesterol, 6.50 (N value 3.63–6.48 mmol/l); triglycerides, 1.37 mmol/l (N value less than 1.7).

Comment Within 48 hours the swelling and marked inflammatory response of the forefoot had resolved.

Question How does peripheral vascular disease in the diabetic differ from that in the non-diabetic?

Answer

1   Peripheral vascular disease is commoner in the diabetic.

2   In the non-diabetic the sex ratio of peripheral vascular disease is Male:Female: 30:1 whereas in the diabetic the ratio is 2:1.

3   In the diabetic multi-segmental occlusions occur associated with diffuse mural changes in between.

4   In the diabetic there is involvement of the collaterals and small blood vessels making surgical correction of the vascular deficiency more difficult.

5   Peripheral vascular disease is more commonly bilateral in the diabetic than the non-diabetic.

6   In the diabetic the most common vessels involved are the anterior and posterior tibial arteries together with the perineal and the more distal vessels. Large and small vessel disease does not necessarily progress at the same rate, thus explaining the presence of tibial pulses in one-third of the patients with established gangrene of the forefoot.

Question What is meant by the term diabetic microangiopathy.

Answer In diabetic microangiopathy thickening of the capillary basement membrane occurs. The degree of thickening increases with the duration of diabetes and may be related to the degree of control over the blood sugar. Such thickening is always greatest in the feet. The precise significance of this change is unknown. It may result in increased permeability of the affected capillaries to both fluid and proteins or limit the escape of leucocytes.

Question What clotting abnormalities have been found in diabetes which may have some influence on the incidence of peripheral vascular disease.

Answer

1   Increased fibrogen level.

2   Decreased fibrinolytic activity.

3   Increased platelet aggregation and adhesiveness.

Question What other factors increase the incidence of gangrene in the diabetic.

Answer

1   Microthrombi form in response to injury adding to the vascular insufficiency.

2   The high blood sugar encourages the development of infection.

3   An associated peripheral neuropathy makes the diabetic

304

unappreciative of pain and, therefore, unaware that minor injuries have taken place

4 Antibiotic penetration of the ischaemic tissues is poor.

Question Following control of the infection what further investigation is required in this patient.

Answer Percutaneous digital vascular imaging.

Question The informative films taken are shown in Figs 31.1 and 31.2. What do these show.

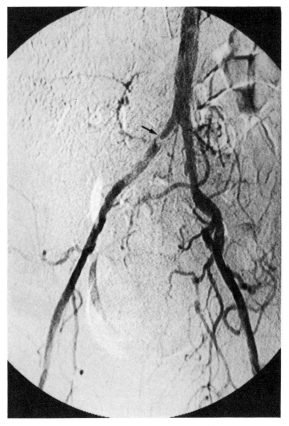

31.1

Answer Figure 31.1 shows the lower end of the aorta and the iliac vessels. Note the localized stricture just distal to the origin of the right common iliac and the absence of the right internal iliac artery. Figure 31.2 shows the extremely poor flow in the lower third of the superficial femoral artery on the right side with reasonable flow on the left.

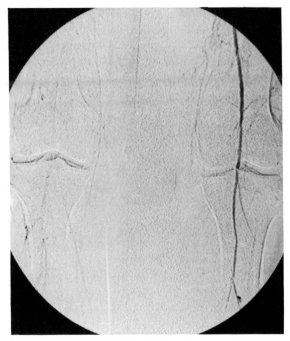

31.2

Question What do the findings in Fig. 31.2 suggest.

Answer That in addition to the stricture at the origin of the common iliac further disease will be present in the superficial femoral probably distal to the origin of the deep femoral, profunda femoris.

Question How would you treat this patient.

Answer The iliac lesion is extremely suitable for percutaneous transluminal balloon angioplasty.

Comment This was performed 10 days after admission.

Question What is the balloon made of.

Answer Polyethylene which has the advantage of retaining its preset dimensions at high inflation pressure with little risk of balloon rupture. Using standard double lumen catheters it allows the insertion of a guide wire, recording of pressure, arteriography and, if necessary, the administration of drugs.

Question How is the technique performed.

Answer The common femoral is cannulated using the Seldinger technique, a local anaesthesia and, if necessary, intravenous Valium.

The proximal intra-arterial pressure is now recorded after which a flexible guidewire is manipulated through the lesion under fluoroscopic control followed by a tapered catheter so that the proximal arteral pressure can be measured.

Comment In this patient, prior to angioplasty, the pressure gradient across the block was 100 mmHg.

The catheter is then exchanged for the appropriate balloon catheter which is then positioned across the stricture and inflated for between 20 and 30 seconds at a pressure of between 4 and 12 atmospheres according to the make and size of the balloon used. This may be repeated several times until the initial balloon deformity is abolished. Thereafter post dilatation angiograms and pressure readings can be made. One important technical point is to keep the guide wire through the lesion at all times.

Question Why is this important.

Answer Because reintroduction of the guide wire following dilatation may lead to dissection if the guide wire passes through the disrupted intima.

Question How long should the patient maintain pressure on the puncture wound.

Answer At least 30 minutes. Even so late 'explosive' bleeding may occur. The blood finding its way to the surface, which is good, or producing a massive haematoma.

Question What medication is recommended by some interventional radiologists following this procedure.

Answer

1 Tolazoline (Priscol, Ciba) 50 mg at the end of the procedure by slow intra-arterial injection to counter any tendency to vasoconstriction.

2 Dipyridamole (Persantin, Bochringer Ingelheim UK). This drug acts as an antithrombotic agent, activating platelet adenylcyclase by the potentiation of endogenous prostacyclin. This drug is administered in a dose of 100 mg tds for say six months.

Comment In this patient the pressure gradient across the stricture was eliminated completely and the right common femoral pulse, initially impalpable became clearly palpable. The distal pulses remained absent, however, although the foot became warmer and perhaps slightly less painful.

Question Following iliac angioplasty what results can be expected.

Answer There is an initial success rate of 90 per cent and in this group of patients patency is maintained in approximately 90 per cent at one year, 85 per cent at two years and 80 per cent at three years. This compares with patency rates achieved by aorto-bifemoral grafting of 95 per cent at one year, 90 per cent at two years and 85 per cent at three years.

Furthermore, the mortality of angioplasty is negligible whereas for reconstructive surgery a mortality of between 2 and 5 per cent can be expected.

Comment Some six days later a prograde cannulation of the proximal right common femoral artery was performed.

The pre-angioplasty arteriogram is shown in Fig. 31.3.

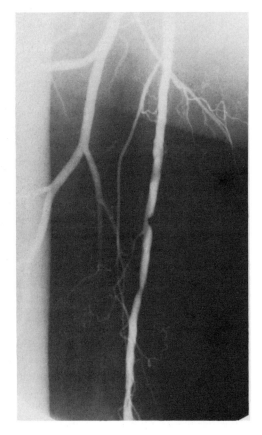

31.3

Question What does this show.

Answer Multiple incomplete strictures in the superficial femoral artery whereas the segment of the deep femoral artery shown appears normal. The small tortuous vessels are collaterals.

Comment Figure 31.4 shows the balloon in place and Fig. 31.5 shows the run off obtained in the popliteal vessel following angioplasty, note the collateral geniculate vessels on the medial side of the knee.

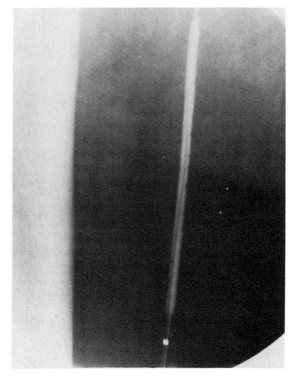

31.4

Question What is the cumulative patency rate following this procedure.

Answer Various authors have reported cumulative patency rates of 80 per cent at one year, 75 per cent at two years and 73 per cent at three years. These results compare favourably with those obtained by bypass vein surgery.

Question What are the chief complications of percutaneous transluminal angioplasty.

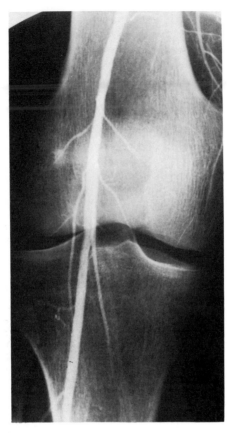

31.5

Answer

    1   At the access site, haemorrhage (experienced by the author himself), haematoma and false aneurysm.

    2   At the site requiring dilatation:

(a) Failure to pass the obstruction and thus failure of the procedure.

(b) Thrombosis.

(c) Embolization.

The presence of complications at the dilatation site nearly always require surgery. Therefore, this procedure should *only* be performed if the services of a competent vascular surgeon are available to the interventional radiologist.

Comment In this patient the fifth toe was amputated through the base of the metatarsal and the fourth through the neck of the metatarsal.

Although the wound was closed; this was a mistake as it soon broke down. Healing occurred slowly by secondary intention and the patient was discharged home three weeks later.

Question Is the prognosis in this patient worse than in the non-diabetic.

Answer Yes. Collected figures show that approximately 40 per cent of diabetics surviving a local amputation are subjected to a major amputation within three years of the initial episode.

Question What is the appearance of a trophic ulcer resulting from peripheral neuropathy.

Answer Trophic ulcers are commonly circular and are surrounded by a large area of hyperkeratosis.

Question How would you treat such a lesion.

Answer The foot should be X-rayed to eliminate osteomyelitis. With no bone involvement the whole area must be deroofed and left to heal by secondary intention. If bone is involved the affected bone has to be removed. The wound should be left open and, if possible, delayed suture should be performed. Assuming there is no proximal large vessel disease, or that large vessel disease has been treated such a wound should heal fairly rapidly as in this case.

32

A Caucasian male aged 62 was admitted complaining of a pale, cold and extremely painful right foot of 6 hours duration. Although the pallor and coldness were of recent onset he had noted some pain in the foot for approximately two days prior to admission, and had observed that even limited walking not only made the pain in the foot worse but also caused a dull ache in the right calf.

Previous medical history Ten years previously a bilateral herniotomy had been performed. For several years he had suffered from chronic bronchitis and emphysema the treatment of which had included aminophylline, 250 mg orally twice daily and a salbutamol sulphate (Ventolin, Allen & Hanbury's) inhaler, usually used three times a day. He had never suffered a myocardial infarct or cerebrovascular accident.

Social habits A widower, he smoked 15–20 cigarettes a day and drank two pints of beer daily as well as four 'shorts'.

Physical examination

Inspection revealed a thin, slightly breathless man with a pallid right forefoot.

Cardiovascular system Heart sounds normal. Peripheral pulses: present in the upper limbs. In the lower limbs all pulses were present in both legs with the exception of the anterior tibial pulses. However, clinically all the pulses in the right lower limb appeared to be somewhat weaker than those on the left including the common femoral. Auscultation revealed a bruit above the right inguinal ligament.

Doppler pressures in the brachial arteries were 160 mmHg, in the posterior tibial artery on the left 180 mmHg and on the right 140 mmHg.

Respiratory system Poor air entry with marked scattered rhonci throughout both lung fields.

Central nervous system No abnormality detected. Examination of the urine, negative.

Question What do the history and the physical signs suggest.

Answer The presence of a partial occlusion of the external iliac artery at its origin followed by an embolic block of the smaller arteries of the foot.

Question How do you arrive at this conclusion.

Answer The presence of a bruit above the inguinal ligament.

Question What is a bruit.

Answer A bruit is an acoustic vibration caused by disturbance of the normal laminar flow. Turbulent non-laminar flow is produced as the blood passes through a stenotic arterial segment into a vessel of normal calibre. A bruit is heard only when a pressure gradient exists across the partially occluded vessel.

Question When is the bruit loudest.

Answer In the early part of systole. However, at rest when only slight stenosis is present, because of the relatively slow rate of blood flow no sound may be heard since the pressure gradient may be negligible. As the stenosis progresses, however, and the pressure gradient increases so the velocity of blood flow across the constriction accelerates producing an audible vibration even at rest which may, in extreme cases, extend into diastole.

Question Is a bruit accentuated by exercise.

Answer Yes. Because even a slight stenosis may significantly retard the increased blood flow produced by exercise whilst at the same time peripheral vasodilatation enhances the rate at which blood flows into the microcirculation thus increasing the pressure gradient at the point of obstruction.

Question Is a bruit present when complete obstruction of the vessel is present.

Answer No. Because of the absence of flow distal to the obstruction.

Question Is it possible to produce an iatrogenic bruit.

Answer Yes, by pressing too hard with the diaphragm of the stethoscope over the artery thus causing deformity of the vessel under examination.

Question Does a bruit necessarily mean that the artery itself is stenosed.

Answer No.

1   The normal laminar flow can be disturbed by dilatation and tortuosity.

2   An arterio-venous fistula is always associated with a bruit.

3   The vessel may be compressed by external forces, e.g. a tumour.

Comment In this case the site of the bruit indicates a partial stenosis in the region of the bifurcation of the common iliac artery. The difference in Doppler pressures between the right and left posterior tibial arteries confirms that the blood flow to the right leg is less than to the left.

Question How is a Doppler ultrasonic flow meter used to determine the blood pressure.

Answer A blood pressure cuff is wrapped around the leg and the pressure in it raised to above systolic level, the Doppler probe is positioned

313

over the posterior tibial artery after which the pressure in the cuff is dropped in stepwise fashion until there is a reappearance of sound over the artery as detected by the probe. The level at which this occurs is considered to be the systolic blood pressure.

Comment The presence of severe pain, the rapid development of coldness and pallor in the right foot together with a palpable posterior tibial pulse indicate that sudden total occlusion of the plantar arteries must have occurred.

Question What might have caused the partial occlusion in the region of the bifurcation of the common iliac artery in this patient.

Answer

1 An arterial embolus.

2 An atheromatous plaque beneath which haemorrhage had occurred or upon which thrombus had formed.

2 A spontaneous arterial thrombosis in a previously normal blood vessel.

The latter can reportedly occur in patients suffering from cardiac arrythmias, the nephrotic syndrome, congestive failure, severe dehydration or prolonged immobilization.

Question Would you consider that the cause of this patient's problem was an arterial embolus.

Answer There can be no doubt that the vascular episode in the foot is embolic in nature. However, some doubt must exist as to pathology in the iliac vessels.

Question Why.

Answer Because:

1 Arterial emboli normally lodge at points of bifurcation producing total occlusion of the involved vessel. In this patient all the physical signs point to an incomplete block of the major vessels.

2 The origin of an arterial embolus is normally evident. Eighty per cent of all emboli formed of clotted material arise from the heart.

All other sources are rare but a peripheral embolus can arise from an aneurysm of the thoracic or abdominal aorta or from thrombi forming on ulcerated atherosclerotic plaques.

Question What cardiac conditions predispose to aseptic peripheral arterial emboli.

Answer

1 Valvular heart disease:

(a) atherosclerotic.

(b) following rheumatic fever.

2 Atrial disorders:

(a) atrial fibrillation: clots form in the left atrium due to incomplete emptying causing stasis.

(b) atrial dilatation caused by mitral stenosis.

3 Myocardial infarction: in 50 per cent of infarcts which involve the endocardium mural clots form on the involved surface. In the majority of patients if embolization is to occur it does so in the first three weeks. Later embolization may occur from a cardiac aneurysm secondary to infarction.

Question Name two rare causes of peripheral arterial embolus.

Answer

1 Fragmentation of an atrial myxoma.

2 Paradoxical embolization; the embolus arising from a thrombus in the deep veins of the lower limbs or pelvis passing upwards to the heart and then into the peripheral arterial system via a patent foramen ovale.

Comment Despite the above arguments it was considered reasonable to explore the right femoral artery. This was done using 50 ml of 0.5 per cent lignocaine hydrochloride (Xylocaine, Astra) with 1:200000 adrenaline as the local anaesthetic.

A vertical groin incision was made and control of the common femoral, superficial femoral and profunda femoris was obtained after which the patient was given 5000 units of heparin intravenously.

An arteriotomy wound was made in the common femoral artery and a No. 3 Fogarty Catheter was passed distally to the level of the ankle with no difficulty. However, on withdrawing the catheter with gradual dilatation of the balloon no thrombus or clot was obtained. Similarly, no solid material was obtained from the profunda femoris.

A No. 5 Fogarty catheter was then passed proximally and a significant increase in flow obtained from the arteriotomy following the extraction of a partially red/partially pale thrombus measuring 8 cm in length and 0.6 cm in diameter (Fig. 32.1). Following this the arteriotomy was closed with No. 5 prolene after which the wound was closed.

At the conclusion of the operation the foot was still cold and white. On the day following operation the patient received Dextran 40 and 5000 units of heparin three times a day, by the subcutaneous route, this regime being continued for three days. On the first post-operative day the administration of warfarin sodium BP was commenced.

Question Give a suitable schedule for warfarin administration.

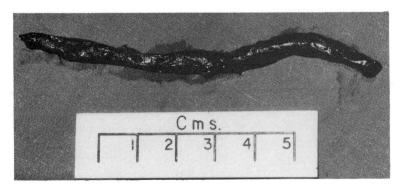

32.1

Answer A loading dose of 10 mg, followed by 5 mg on successive days. On the third day the prothrombin time should be checked and the daily dose thereafter recommended according to the result.

Comment In this patient the prothrombin time on the third day of administration was 58 seconds thus greatly exceeding the normally accepted therapeutic level of 2.5 times the normal. After various modifications of the dose over the succeeding eight days it appeared that a daily dose of 2 mg would probably be sufficient to achieve a satisfactory therapeutic result.

Question What is the major adverse effect of warfarin.
Answer Bleeding, usually adequately controlled by discontinuing the drug and administering by mouth or by slow intravenous injection between 2 and 20 mg of phytomenadione.

Comment On the second post-operative day digital vascular imaging was performed, the radiographs being obtained by the injection of an intravenous bolus of 165 ml of Niopam 3 into the right atrium by a catheter introduced via the right basilic vein.

The intravenous route was used because the patient was anticoagulated. The results are shown in Figs 32.2, 32.3 and 32.4.

Question What do these figures show?
Answer Common, superficial femoral and profunda femoris arteries of good and uniform diameter. A normal trifurcation in the popliteal region with apparently normal anterior and posterior tibial arteries together with a normal peroneal artery.

However, the anterior tibial artery tapers to an end at the lower

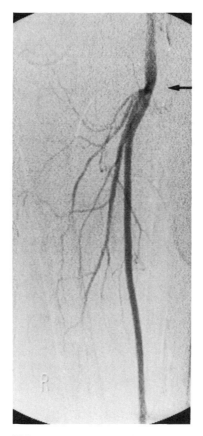

32.2

third of the tibia and both the posterior, tibial and peroneal arteries can only be identified to the level of the ankle joint.

Question What conclusion do you draw.

Answer That distal small vessel occlusion had occurred and that there appears to be no evidence of atherosclerosis in the major vessels of the lower limb.

Comment It became increasingly obvious that the toes were becoming gangrenous and in order to attempt to limit this process a lumbar sympathectomy was performed.

Question How can this be accomplished.

Answer Surgical sympathectomy is now only rarely performed. More commonly the sympathetic outflow to the lower limb is destroyed

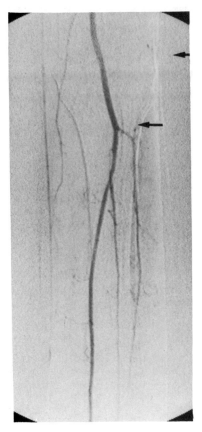

32.3

by the injection of 5 per cent phenol into the lumbar sympathetic ganglia.

Question In which root do the preganglionic fibres pass to reach the sympathetic trunk.

Answer In the ventral nerve roots as medulated fibres which on leaving the respective roots form the white rami communicantes which synapse in the various ganglia of the sympathetic trunk.

Question From what segments of the spinal cord do sympathetic fibres arise.

Answer From the first thoracic to the second lumbar segments.

Question Which ganglia must be destroyed in order to effectively destroy the sympathetic supply to the lower limb.

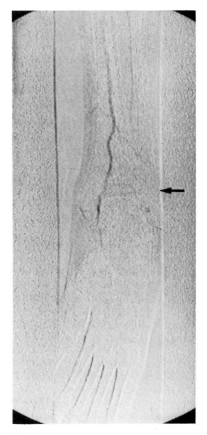

32.4

Answer The second, third and fourth lumbar ganglia.

Question How is a chemical sympathectomy performed.

Answer Three 15 cm, 18 gauge needles are required, each needle being marked at 10 cm from the point.

The patient is placed into the lateral position and each needle is inserted 7.5 cm lateral to the spinous processes of the lumbar vertebrae on a level with the cephalic borders of the second, third and fourth lumbar vertebrae. If each needle is inserted at right angles to the skin the point of the needle will strike the body of the appropriate lumbar vertebra at a depth of 10 cm. If a bony obstruction is encountered prior to 10 cm it will be a transverse process.

Having located the body of the vertebra the needle is withdrawn, re-angulated and reinserted aiming to graze the body of the vertebra arresting its advance at 10 cm in a thin and 12 cm in a fat stocky individual.

Two or three ml of one per cent lignocaine are then injected into each needle and if this is followed by venous dilatation in the lower limb and foot it can be assumed that the position of the needles is correct. Thereafter 2–3 ml of five per cent phenol is injected into each needle. In hospitals with the necessary equipment this procedure can be carried out using an image intensifier.

Question What complications can occur.

Answer

1 The patient might complain of severe pains in the distribution of the second, third and fourth lumbar nerve roots. This normally disappears within a few days.

2 Temporary psoas weakness may occur.

Question What is accomplished by lumbar sympathectomy.

Answer An initial marked increase in the cutaneous blood flow occurs which lasts only a short time. Thereafter a small augmentation persists, less than double the pre-sympathectomy reading.

Comment In this patient little obvious clinical benefit was achieved and morphine (MST) was required to control pain.

Question In this patient the posterior tibial pulse was present and gangrene was developing in the forefoot only, what amputation would you advise.

Answer This represented the ideal situation in which to perform a Syme's amputation.

Question What is the advantage of a Syme's amputation.

Answer When healed, it produces a weight bearing stump.

Question Are there any disadvantages.

Answer The only disadvantage is its cosmetic appearance since any prosthesis must accommodate the flair of the distal tibial metaphysis which is covered by the heavy plantar skin.

Comment The amputation healed satisfactorily (Fig. 32.5) and the question now arose as to whether this patient should be continued on anticoagulant therapy. It was decided that this depended on the condition of the aorta and the iliac vessels, since if thrombosis had recurred at the seat of an athermatous plaque it would be necessary to continue anticoagulant therapy whereas if the vessels appeared to be normal in the absence of any demonstrable cardiac lesion there would be little value in continued medication.

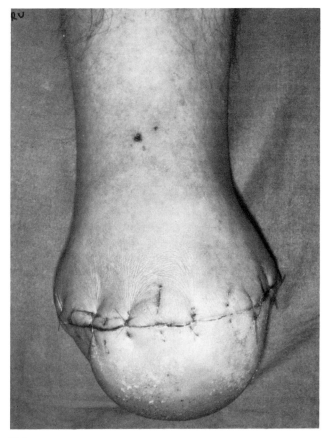

32.5

Therefore, prior to making a decision it was decided to perform a
further digital vascular imaging of the aorta and its chief branches.
In order to do this the anticoagulants were reversed and the 16th
post-operative day a second DVI was carried out.

These showed a normal vascular tree and it was, therefore, decided
to discontinue anticoagulants. When last seen nine months later the
patient was in reasonable health and was well satisfied with his
amputation.

33

A Caucasian male age 72 was admitted because of the incidental finding of a large pulsating swelling in the abdomen during the course of investigation for difficulty of micturition and nocturia.

Previous medical history Eighteen years previously he had been seen complaining of claudication in the right calf after walking approximately 300 yards. At that time he admitted to smoking 20 cigarettes a day. His BP was 160/100. Abdominal examination negative. Examination of the peripheral pulses in the lower limbs revealed both common femoral pulses present but no distal pulses were palpable. A diagnosis of bilateral femoro-popliteal blocks was made but in view of the fact that he could perform his work and sleep without difficulty no active treatment was advised but he was advised to cease smoking and the work's doctor placed him on the drug Atromid-S.

Question What is clofibrate and what is its theoretical use in peripheral vascular disease.

Answer Clofibrate is chlorophenoxyisobutyrate, an ester rapidly converted to an acid in the body. Administered in a dose of 20–30 mg/kg daily in three divided doses it is effective in reducing the concentrations of endogenous triglycerides and VLDL (very low density lipoprotein). It can be expected to lower plasma triglyceride concentrations by about 20 per cent but it is less effective in lowering the serum cholesterol. The mechanism of action of this drug is unknown. One hypothesis is that it has a direct effect on the liver, exerting a major effect on the synthesis and/or secretion of hepatic very low density lipoproteins. It is the treatment of choice of Type III hyperlipoproteinaemia. However, its influence of the overall mortality in coronary artery disease is disappointing. One can, therefore, assume that it is probably ineffective in preventing or reversing the development of atherosclerosis affecting the peripheral vascular system.

Comment After several months his claudication distance increased and at the time of his admission he no longer found any difficulty in walking up to 800 yards.

Question Why has the claudication distance increased.

Answer Because of the development of collaterals.

Question What vessels form the collateral circulation when the superficial femoral artery is occluded.

Answer Collateral circulation is established through the profunda femoris or one of its principal branches augmented by branches of the medial or lateral circumflex femoral arteries which communicate with the highest medial and lateral genicular arteries.

Comment In this patient examination of the films taken in the course of an intravenous pyelogram revealed lateral displacement of the ureters.

Question What conditions will produce lateral displacement of the ureter.

Answer Any retroperitoneal swelling of sufficient size, e.g. an aneurysm of the aorta, para-aortic lymph node enlargement.

Physical examination This revealed no abnormality in any system other than a palpable expansile pulsatory mass in the abdomen and absent anterior and posterior tibial pulses in the right leg.

Question What is the diagnosis.

Answer An aneurysm of the abdominal aorta.

Question Can any other form of pulsating tumour be found in the abdomen.

Answer Any mass overlying the aorta will give rise to a transmitted pulsation. Transmitted and expansile are easily distinguished on physical examination.

Question What types of aneurysm are recognized.

Answer

1 Fusiform, spindle-like dilatations.

2 Saccular, asymmetrical dilatations.

3 Dissecting, caused by an intimal tear allowing blood to leak into the area between the intima and media.

4 False, a complete tear of the arterial wall may, if not rapidly closed, permit the extravasation of blood into the tissue surrounding the vessel. If the tear is not sealed a periarterial pulsating haematoma forms.

5 Arterio-venous, due to the formation of an arterio-venous fistula.

6 Cirsoid, a mass of dilated, pulsating serpinginous vessels, usually associated with a congenital arteriovenous shunt.

Question What is the commonest cause of aneurysmal dilatation.

Answer Atherosclerosis, due to the gradual destruction of the media.

Question A common radiological physical sign of an abdominal aneurysm is shown in Fig. 33.1. What is it.

Answer Calcification.

Question Figure 33.2 is a subtraction film following digital vascular imaging of an aortic aneurysm. What does it show.

Answer It shows the outline of the aneurysm and the column of contrast

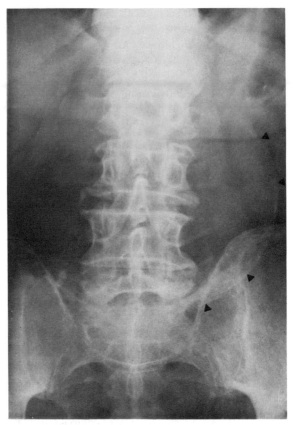

33.1

medium passing in a somewhat eccentric manner through the sac.

Question Why is the contrast column not filling the whole of the aneurysmal sac.

Answer Because thrombus and clot formation occur within the lumen. The mixed thrombus/clot removed from within the aneurysm in the patient described is shown in Fig. 33.3.

Question Is thrombosis and clotting within an aneurysm of clinical importance.

Answer Yes. At any time fragmentation may occur causing emboli which impacting distally may cause peripheral vascular obstruction. In the upper limb small emboli from a subclavian aneurysm may be a cause of Raynaud's phenomenon.

Question What causes, other than atherosclerosis, lead to the development of aneurysms.

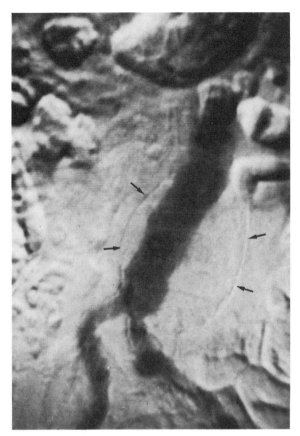

33.2

Answer

1 Acute infection leading to the formation of a mycotic aneurysm.

2 Chronic infection; syphilis. Infection with the *Treponema pallidum* results in obstruction of the vasa vasorum due to intimal proliferation. This leads to impaired nutrition and weakness of the wall of the affected vessel. Syphilitic aneurysms most commonly involve the ascending aorta, possibly due to the rich lymphatic network in this area.

3 Inherited connective tissue defects:

(a) Marfan's syndrome (Arachnodactyly). This disease, inherited as a dominant trait, causes defects in the connective tissue in many parts of the body. The limbs grow to extraordinary lengths and the fingers are long and spidery. Other skeletal defects associated with

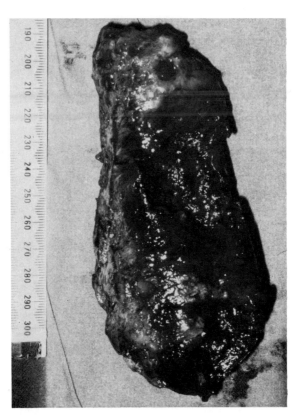

33.3

the condition are a high palatal arch, kyphoscoliosis, spondyl-
olisthesis, slipped epiphyses, long unstable feet and osteoporosis.
Medial mucoid degeneration of the ascending aorta leads to widening
of the aortic valve ring and aortic regurgitation. A split in the intima
allows the development of a dissecting aneurysm.

(b) Ehlers-Danlos syndrome (hyperelastosis cutis). This is also an
autosomal dominant trait in which a defect in collagen metabolism
occurs. The most characteristic feature is a thin, hyperplastic, brittle
and fragile skin. Medial mucoid degeneration again predisposes to
the development of dissecting aneurysms of the arch of the aorta.

4   Post stenotic dilatations, seen most commonly in the third part
of the subclavian artery distal to the point at which it crosses a
cervical rib.

5   Anastomotic aneurysms; such aneurysms are really pulsating
haematomata, false aneurysms, occurring at suture lines where a

graft joins an artery. They are more common following the use of prosthetic grafts than autogenous vein grafts and they are more common following end to side than end to end anastomoses.

6 Congenital. Normally called congenital but never present at birth are the Berry aneurysms occurring on the circle of Willis. These are the result of defects in the media. Such defects constitute distinct weaknesses, particularly in the circle of Willis where the vessels lie unsupported in the subarachnoid space.

Question What are the presenting symptoms associated with abdominal aneurysms.

Answer

1 As in this patient the aneurysm may be silent.

2 The patient may have observed a pulsating swelling in the abdomen.

3 Localized abdominal pain may be felt due to expansion of the sac.

4 Erosion of the bodies of the lumbar vertebra may lead to backache.

5 Embolic phenomena may lead to examination.

6 Rupture (see below).

Question In this patient the presence of the aneurysm was first noted on an intravenous pyelogram; what ureteric abnormalities may occur in the presence of an abdominal aneurysm.

Answer

1 The ureters may be displaced laterally.

2 The ureters may be drawn inwards towards the midline. This occurs only if organization of a retroperitoneal haematoma has occurred.

3 Ureteric obstruction is occasionally observed, the result of retroperitoneal inflammation rather than external pressure.

Question Can the majority of aortic aneurysms be treated surgically.

Answer Yes. Whilst there may be some fusiform dilatation of the aorta above the origin of the aneurysm in the great majority of cases abdominal aneurysms arise below the origin of the renal arteries.

Question What is the commonest complication associated with an aortic aneurysm.

Answer Rupture, this usually leads to a massive retroperitoneal haematoma followed by the rapid development of hypovolaemic shock. However, rupture may also occur into the peritoneal cavity, or very rarely into the duodenum or inferior vena cava.

Question What symptoms would be associated with rupture into the duodenum.

Answer A haematemesis, the severity of which will be determined by the size of the rupture. The author was once playing bridge with an elderly general practitioner in the south position when he said he felt faint and nauseated. He left the bridge table and had a small vomit. Some minutes later he left the table again with the same symptoms. Somewhat concerned he was asked what he was vomiting. His reply was, 'not to worry, it's only the bottle of red wine I had for lunch'. He died some seven days later.

Question What situation follows rupture into the inferior vena cava.

Answer High output heart failure associated with grossly swollen legs.

Question What is the mortality associated with the resection of an uncomplicated abdominal aneurysm.

Answer Approximately 5 per cent.

Question What is the mortality associated with resection following rupture.

Answer Mortality is related to the condition of the patient at the time of operation and the expertise of the surgeon. Thus in reasonably competent hands the mortality may be as low as 50 per cent.

Question What is the prognosis following successful resection.

Answer Providing the patient does not suffer from ischaemic heart disease or hypertension life expectancy is virtually normal.

Question What specific investigation is essential in a patient suffering from an asymptomatic abdominal aneurysm.

Answer Ultrasonography. This determines the diameter of the aneurysm.

Question Why is this information important.

Answer Because the risk of rupture increases rapidly once the aneurysm reaches 6–7 cm in diameter.

Comment In this patient the aneurysmal size, as measured by ultrasonography, was 5.4 cm (Fig. 33.4), i.e. approaching the critical diameter. However, when taking the history this patient declared that he was a Jehovah's witness and that he refused to contemplate any blood transfusion. In fact even blood drawn into syringe from a peripheral vein should not be reintroduced into the circulation. This excludes one from taking one or two units prior to surgery and using them during the operation.

A decision was made after considerable debate that he should undergo surgery since the aneurysm had almost reached a critical size and undoubtedly if rupture occurred death was inevitable.

Question Who was the first surgeon to successfully resect an abdominal aortic aneurysm.

Answer Dubost in 1952.

Question Is the affected segment of the aorta excised.

Answer No. Following the administration of 5000 units of heparin control of the aorta above and below the aneurysm is obtained and the sac

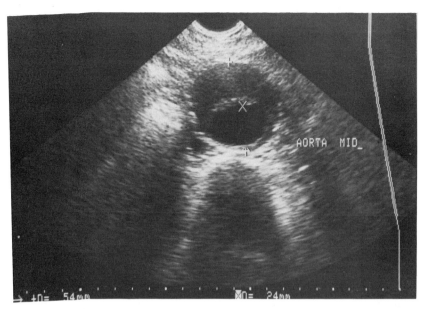

AORTA MID

→ +0= 54mm   X0= 24mm

33.4

is incised longitudinally. The lumbar vessels are now controlled by stitches placed from within the aorta after which a preclotted knitted Dacron graft, appropriate in diameter and length is sutured in place. A tube graft should be cut to such a length that when sutured in place it will be under moderate tension.

Question What early complications may follow excision of an aortic aneurysm.

Answer Haemorrhage, thrombosis, emboli, ileus, post-operative ischaemia of the lower sigmoid due to division in the inferior mesenteric artery.

Comment This patient underwent the successful excision of his abdominal aneurysm without the use of blood. He was given, during the course of the operation, 1000 ml of Hartmann's solution and 1500 ml of haemaccel. Seen nine months after operation he was symptom free.

List of viva topics